"The research described in this book would not have been possible without the generous support of the Medical Research Council, UK, the University of Cambridge and University College London."

The Developing Visual Brain

JANETTE ATKINSON

Visual Development Unit
University College London

OXFORD PSYCHOLOGY SERIES
NO. 32

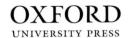

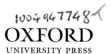

OXFORD

UNIVERSITY PRESS

Great Clarendon Street, Oxford OX2 6DP

Oxford University Press is a department of the University of Oxford.
It furthers the University's objective of excellence in research, scholarship,
and education by publishing worldwide in

Oxford New York

Auckland Bangkok Buenos Aires Cape Town Chennai
Dar es Salaam Delhi Hong Kong Istanbul Karachi Kolkata
Kuala Lumpur Madrid Melbourne Mexico City Mumbai Nairobi
São Paulo Shanghai Singapore Taipei Tokyo Toronto

and an associated company in Berlin

Oxford is a registered trade mark of Oxford University Press
in the UK and in certain other countries

Published in the United States
by Oxford University Press Inc., New York

© Janette Atkinson 2000

A catalogue record for this book is available from the British Library

Library of Congress Cataloging in Publication Data
Atkinson, Janette
The developing visual brain/ Janette Atkinson.
Oxford psychology series ; no. 32)
Includes bibliographical references and index.
1. Visual perception in infants.   2. Vision in infants.   I. Title.   II. Series.
BF720.V57 A85 2000   155.42'2214—dc21   99-056762

ISBN 0 19 852297 5 (Hbk)
ISBN 0 19 852599 0 (Pbk)

Typeset by J&L Composition Ltd,
Filey, North Yorkshire
Printed in Great Britain
on acid-free paper by
TJ International, Padstow

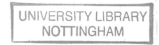

Preface

Our work with infants started in the Cambridge Physiological Laboratory, where I was working with Fergus Campbell as a relatively new postdoctoral student. Fergus had the usual stream of prestigious visitors and international colleagues working with him, as well as his many local colleagues including John Robson, Colin Blakemore, Horace Barlow and Roger Carpenter and their graduate students such as Tony Movshon, Peter Lennie, Dave Tolhurst, and Donald Macleod. Serendipitously for us, one such visitor was Alan Hein who gave a talk in the Craik Laboratory in the spring of 1973. I was in the last months of pregnancy with our first child and was already planning some infant psychophysics to measure contrast sensitivity, using adaptations of adult methods and Fourier analysis. On relating these ideas to Alan he told me about Davida Teller's new adaptation of Fantz's preferential looking paradigm, which Davida called 'forced-choice preferential looking'. Apparently, Davida was developing this method for testing infants. I wrote to Davida, who kindly sent me a pre-print of the method. Ol and I set to getting ready to run the first infant contrast sensitivity test with our first child, Fleur.

There was no concept of 'maternity leave' in the University of Cambridge at that time ('academic ladies usually arrange their births in the long vacation'—quote from the appropriately called 'Old Schools' of Cambridge University). Consequently, I worked in the lab up to the evening before Fleur was born and returned a few weeks later with her in my arms to start testing. With the generosity and collaboration which perfused the Craik lab at that time, we arranged a time-share of the experimental equipment with Tony Movshon (then working with Colin Blakemore): Tony would run mainly in the daytime, we would run in the evening and night—a mixture of cigarette butts and nappies causing mutual disgust on both sides!

In the first 3 months of Fleur's life we lived in the lab—it was probably the most careful and dedicated infant study we have ever undertaken. We were very new to babies and to the quirks of testing infants and we had to be sure that our results were reliable and sensible. Hence every point of the meagre contrast sensitivity functions we produced was estimated many times. If Fleur was fretty or sleepy the data were discarded.

We published the results in *Nature,* recognizing the debt that we owed to Davida Teller (whose name we did offer to put on the paper, but she was too modest). As a mild academic joke, we put Fleur's name on the paper as the third author. This had rather serious repercussions when there was an invitation from Professor Van der Tweel in Amsterdam to attend a Dutch meeting to talk about our preliminary studies on infants. The invitation was to Oliver and Fleur Braddick. Ol complicated the situation further by ringing the Dutch lab to say that Fleur Braddick would not be accompanying him to the meeting but rather Janette Atkinson, his colleague, would be with him and that he would like to book a double room in the hotel for himself and Dr Atkinson. Moral outrage at the Dutch end, thinking that Ol must be deserting his wife, Fleur, to travel, a deux, with his research colleague Janette Atkinson, almost caused our invitation to be cancelled. Fortunately Dick Cavonius, working in the Dutch lab at the time and being at an advanced state of knowledge concerning relationships in Cambridge, explained who Fleur Braddick was, and her age. Because of all this, I am afraid that our three other children have only been acknowledged on their infant publications, rather than having full authorship.

Ambitious as ever, we started a second study of perception of vertical and horizontal symmetry with Fleur. This was never completed owing to the apparatus flying into the motorway bushes from the top of our ancient Volvo, as we attempted to lose no testing time by taking the set-up to my parent's home in the North for Christmas. Similar results to those we found in this study were published by Mark Bornstein in 1985.

After our attempts with Fleur, our second infant study was almost our most ambitious ever. We went to work in Brown University jointly with Lew Lipsitt and Lorrin Riggs in the summer of 1974 for a 3-month period—part of the time we would measure visual evoked potentials (VEPs) within half fields with adult albinos (to investigate their curious decussation of the optic tract) and part of the time we would set up and run a study of stereopsis using the method of sucking habituation (already cleverly adapted and used by Lew Lipsitt, Charles Crook, and Trygg Engen). In such a small time period it was obvious that one or other study would not be completed, and in fact the albino study was not completed because measuring VEPs in one or other half field in albinos (often with accompanying strabismus, eccentric fixation, and nystagmus) turned out to be very difficult, giving rather variable responses even in co-operative adults. (We did get some preliminary results which I am afraid remain in our lab books unpublished.) However, the study on onset of stereopsis in infants was completed in Brown and published in *Perception*, a new journal at that time.

Lew Lipsitt was a tough infant lab director, but taught us a great deal about setting up and running 'an infant facility'. As many of his studies took place in an orphanage run by nuns, he explained to us how important it was for infant researchers to be seen as representatives of responsible paediatric science, explaining their experimental paradigms to people outside science and behaving with decorum. We remember a memo sent round by Lew stating that all infant researchers should 'wear clean lab coats, their hair should be tied back and that no one should wear 'play' clothes or trainers in the infant lab or orphanage'. We had to be there at 6.30 a.m. to test infants before their breakfast and bath. He was an excellent model leader (and indeed excellent yo-yo-ist as well), although I have rarely been able to match his discipline with dress code for people in our own lab. The infant lab in the Roman Catholic orphanage was very well run by the nuns and was extremely disciplined and peaceful. The summer in Lew's infant lab has several fairly funny memories for me, I think the best was a comment from one of the nuns who, discovering that one of Lew's researchers was Roman Catholic, said 'well it may not make any difference to your life now in testing babies, but you'll be glad of your religion when you get to heaven'. There obviously wasn't much hope for the rest of us in her eyes, either testing babies on earth or afterwards.

When we returned to Cambridge we set up the *Infant Perception Study* in rooms in 28 Trumpington Street, some of which were kindly 'lent' to us by Horace Barlow. As well as our experience in Brown, we also toured may of the active infant labs at that time—Tom Bower, Colwyn Trevarthen, Harry McGurk, Michael Lewis, Jerome Kagan, and Phil Salapatek. At that time there were a few other groups about to set up infant vision psychophysics: one in Davida Teller's lab; one in Dick Held's in MIT, and another by Phil Salapatek in Minneapolis with Marty Banks and Dick Aslin as new researchers. Our lab was completed a few weeks before Hugo, our second child, was born. The house was an old hospital residency, virtually unconverted by the University. I can remember repainting the rather dingy bathroom, but because I was such an odd shape at the time was unable to bend down to paint the wall under the wash-bowl! Fortunately, we had collected two willing researchers—Ian Bushnell and Kathie Moar—and together the four of us got the bathroom finished before Hugo was born and the 'Baby Lab', as it has since been called, got started.

The first studies with Hugo were on contrast sensitivity in the first few months of life. We started to learn how to measure visual evoked potentials in babies, to be able to compare the results with behavioural preferential looking methods. Hugo was one of the first 'volunteers' for the new baby lab and was the 'active participant' at 6 months of age in our study (together with Laurence Harris) comparing his and my contrast sensitivity function. To keep Hugo's attention we used an 'active face super-imposed on the grating pattern' (so the paper reads). In actual fact this was Ol, Laurence, and I dancing round, complete with maracas, singing every song in our repertoire—the favourite for Hugo at the time being 'Concrete and Clay'. Following this study we moved on to newborns, and arranged to test them in the Cambridge Maternity Hospital. For the first week of testing we were unable to record a single significant pattern VEP—we couldn't understand it after our success with slightly older infants. In despair I discussed it with Fergus who sent me off to the EEG Department in the hospital to find out how they did it. It turns out that newborns are covered in a somewhat oily cling-wrap for the first few days after birth and have rather high skin resistance unless the skin is cleaned well before placement of the surface electrodes. We learnt from them how to rub a little harder and to record VEPs successfully in newborns.

After this the group grew and grew. Lorrin, our third child, heralded the advent of photorefraction—in fact he was photorefracted a few hours after birth in the maternity hospital, when *Mrs Janette Braddick* (in dressing gown) went missing from the postnatal ward and miraculously changed into white-coated *Dr Janette Atkinson*. In the dayroom at the end of the ward Howard Howland, our wonderfully tolerant new colleague and co-inventor with his brother of photorefraction, amiably jumped up and down with Christmas lights on his head in a wild attempt to get Lorrin—even then appearing coolly laid back—to focus on him behind the camera. It worked and by a serendipitous misfocusing of the camera on our part, we discovered a new method called 'isotropic photorefraction', for refracting young infants. After this success with babies we tried infant monkeys in Torsten Wiesel's lab and even adult monkeys with Alan Cowey in Oxford. The latter was a hilarious session, especially as monkeys, unlike humans, hate eye to eye contact—at one stage a huge bunch of bananas was madly waved above the camera, in the hope of getting them to look at the camera. We tried getting them to attend by turning all the lights off in the room except for a lamp illuminating the bananas, and eventually got their attention when one of the experimenters stumbled over the lead from the lamp in the dark, accompanied by a lot of swearing and background noise of crashing apparatus! In the end we realized that the monkeys were trained to fixate steadily in the discrimination apparatus and of course this was the best way to test them.

Around this time we made two short successful research visits: one to New York and one to Boston. In New York, once again Tony Movshon came up trumps by rescuing us from the hell of North Terminal in JFK airport at 2 a.m. with a young baby (Lorrin), who had just managed to get us rapidly through immigration by choking on a boiled sweet. Tony not only found us paper towels in his car to clean up the choking child and mother, but also drove us to an apartment he had found for us. I was impressed by Tony's resourcefulness, cheerfulness, and tolerance of children under the circumstances, but he informed me that it was all part of the training as an electrophysiologist—where one often had to be adaptive and resilient in messy situations in the middle of the night. Besides Tony and his wife Meg, our stay in New York would not have been at all possible without the hospitality of Louise Hainline. Part way through our stay, the apartment in NYC which we were renting suddenly needed to be repossessed by the owners. Louise took into her home in Brooklyn the entire Braddick/Atkinson tribe (nine of us including many children, two Grandmothers, and an aupair!) for a month. I don't think Louise's two cats ever recovered from the trauma, but Louise took it all in her stride and even said she enjoyed having us stay.

Our reason for visiting New York was the invitation of Bela Julesz, who decided that, as we were one of the few groups who had successfully recorded VEPs with infants at this time, we might be able to measure development of binocularity in infants using his newly devised dynamic random dot correlogram stimuli. We ran the tests with the much needed help of Ivan Bodis-Wollner and Edwin Raab in Mount Sinai Hospital (later to be the setting in the film *Kramer versus Kramer*, where it is very accurately depicted as a manic all-American hospital on 35 floors, overflowing with patients and emergency rooms). To set up the equipment a vital piece of equipment, a plotter, was kindly lent to us by John Krauskopf from Bell Labs, who brought it into the hospital for us. Unfortunately, on trying to leave the hospital to return the plotter at the end of our stay, we were apprehended and held in custody by armed guards, who were convinced we were stealing hospital property! We were fortunately rescued by telephone calls to Ivan and Bela.

Our other visit was to MIT, where Ol worked with David Marr and we both worked in Dick Held's lab. I had already found an interesting transient asymmetry in young infants' optokinetic eye movements back in Cambridge in the previous months. In Boston I extended these studies to both American human babies and infant monkeys. We are particularly indebted to Torsten Wiesel and Dick Held for making the whole project possible and to Joe Bauer for having such a wide ranging set of technical and ethological skills that enabled us to get reliable results from minute macaques.

Our stay in MIT, will probably be remembered by most for the wild English lunch party which we threw, in collusion with Jeremy Wolfe. This event culminated in the whole lab (rather drunk by this time) randomly decorating a very large black drum with small white sticky dots. Its purpose was to enable Jeremy to run experiments on adult human optokinetic motion after-effects. We knew that decorating the drum by ourselves would take days and be extremely boring—however, as a 'party happening' it worked well.

Shortly after Boston we started to make regular summer visits to California. It started as a house exchange with Donald Macleod and Mary Hayhoe, but developed into a regular teaching and research visit (plus some sun and beach of course!). We have many good friends and colleagues there, with Don and Andi Macleod heading the list as being the faithful custodians of all our children's 'Californian necessities' like boogie boards—not too mention accommodating members of our family on numerous occasions. We also thank Jean and George Mandler, Tony and Diana Deutsch, Joan Stiles, Liz Bates, Rama and Diane Ramachandran, Ursula Bellugi, Ed Klima and Terry Sejnowski. One memorable visit was to work in the Salk Institute where we had the audacity to introduce visual psychophysics into Francis Crick's lab. It was a most inspiring time (if a little unnerving for normal human beings like myself in attempting to defend research ideas with Francis). Fortunately, Odile Crick always provided a calming European influence on our visits by inviting us to dinner and showing us her beautiful paintings.

There then followed a 10-year period back in Cambridge in which many collaborators came and went, the baby lab team changed and moved house and we became more established as a serious developmental vision group. However, when Ione was born in September 1988 we decided to go right back to the beginning to measures of contrast sensitivity, but do it even better in terms of comparison techniques and stimuli. This time we ran night and day for every available session with her. She loved the night (and so far still does) and so taxed us by being particularly good for testing at 3 a.m., like many babies. At Christmas we were exhausted and decided to call it a day—the results come later in this book.

Throughout our developmental research we have always had a strong bias towards studies of abnormal human development as well as normal development. Our clinical studies have had three branches: one liaising with ophthalmology and optometry; one with paediatricians and paediatric neurologists; and one with educationalists. Under developmental ophthalmology we have studied development of children with congenital cataracts, strabismus, abnormal refractive errors, amblyopia, and more recently infant glaucoma. Our research, particularly in developing assessment methods for infants, started because of the strong collaboration between the University Departments in Cambridge and the Ophthalmology Department in Addenbrookes Hospital, with Fergus Campbell, Colin Blakemore, and ophthalmologist Peter Watson. We have moved on from studying individual infants with strabismus and amblyopia to devising two large Cambridge Health District Vision Screening programmes, using isotropic photo and videorefraction—a technique we developed especially for infants in collaboration with Howard and Brad Howland from the States. Our screening programmes have also been extended to five other centres in Europe, organized and co-ordinated by the Visual Development Unit, with the centres being led by Francois Vital Durand in Lyon, Mario Angi in Padua, Orlando Alves da Silva in Lisbon, Alfonso Castanera in Barcelona, and Ruxandra Sireteanu in Frankfurt. Collaborating across Europe has been an invigorating experience, and certainly made us more positive about European Unity in the future!

We also had extensive support and collaboration with members of the Department of Paediatrics in Cambridge, in particular Cliff Roberton and John Davis. Their help enabled us to be the first group to measure pattern VEPs for measures of acuity, contrast sensitivity, and binocularity in newborns. We also developed links with Mike Prendergast and Chris Verity in the Child Development Centre and started assessing vision in children with multiple disorders including vision, rather than isolated vision problems. Over the years we have developed links with many paediatric departments and special child assessment units, studying vision in a wide range of children with paediatric problems, including Down syndrome, cerebral palsy, Williams syndrome, autism, and different types and degrees of brain abnormality. This work has led to our current collaborations in London with paediatric teams in University College and the Hammersmith Hospitals. We have been extremely fortunate in finding enthusiasm for our work in many special schools and foundations— for example, those linked to Scope (Meldreth Manor), King's College School Special Unit for Dyslexia, and the Williams Syndrome Foundation. With educationalists we have looked at some aspects of vision in children with learning difficulties, including dyslexia, and started to think about both assessment and training schemes for children with visual and spatial problems.

In 1993, 20 years after we had started our infant studies, we decided to move our main research base to University College. We now have two parts to the Visual Development Unit (VDU)—one in London and one in Cambridge. The old, much loved Cambridge Unit has had to move house twice in the last 5 years, but is now running well, following up several hundred children until they are 6 years with multiple measures of visual, language, visuocognitive, and motor development as part of our Infant Vision Screening programme. In London, the VDU has a diverse range of research activities from studies on infants detecting illusory contours and motion coherence, to toddlers reaching and grabbing toys, to children with perinatal brain damage making amazing recoveries of visual development and to Williams syndrome children telling us about exotic makes of lawn mowers rather than attending to moving visual patterns on computer screens. We are now undertaking some adult research studies looking at vision in adult dyslexic students and functional magnetic resonance imaging analysis of adults looking at the same stimuli we are showing to babies and children, so that we can start to make comparative measures of brain plasticity in development and adulthood.

Most of the work discussed in this book has been done in collaboration with other members of the VDU. Much of the VDU's research contribution is due to Ol Braddick, John Wattam-Bell, and Shirley Anker. There are all the other past and present members who have made very significant contributions to the group's research effort and should be mentioned and thanked by me. They are (in time order), Ian Bushnell, Kathy Moar, Jennifer French, Lesley Ayling, Liz Pimm-Smith, Jackie Day, Jan Vincent, Roseanne Hall, Hilary Stobart, Carol Evans, Bruce Hood, Frank Weeks,

Nicky Gardner, Francoise Mathieu, Joss Smith, Claire Towler, Ann McIntyre, Val Norris, Annette Landy, Kim Durden, Jo Pritchard, Roslyn Hedges, Jo Tricklebank, Sarah Rae, Fiona Macpherson, Bill Bobier, Jonathan Pointer, Mike Nicholls, Claire Hughes, Jackie Wade, David Ehrlich, Louise Nokes, John King, Tom Hartley, Jackie Andrew, Rachel Andrew, Alice Wuensche, Alexandra Mason, Will Curran, Karen Wyatt, Eugenio Mercuri, Justin O'Brien, Chris Newman, Leena Haataja, Andrea Guzzetta, Jon Fowler, Enrico Biagioni, Katrina Richards, and Marko Nardini.

Besides those in the Unit, and those I have already acknowledged above, there is a long list of friends and colleagues who have helped us over the years. Listed in approximate date order they are Stuart Anstis, Fergus and Helen Campbell, Richard Gregory, John Robson, Colin Blakemore, Peter Lennie, John Davis, Cliff Roberton, John Lee, Mike Morgan, Dorothy Einon, Peter and Karen Thompson, Ray Over, David Allen, Michael Mair, Chris Verity, Donald and Mary Broadbent, Tom Troscianko, Lamberto Maffei, Adriana Florentini, Horace, Miranda (and Oscar) Barlow, Peter and Ann Watson, David Healey, Mike Stryker, Alan Cowey, Denis Pelli, John Duncan, Velma Dobson, Joe Bauer, David Marr, Al Yonas, Marty Banks, Dick Aslin, Jackie Van Hof, Janet Rennie, Concetta Morrone and David Burr, Janet Rennie, Ursula Bellugi and Ed Klima, Terry Sejnowski, John Lee, Joan Stiles, Liz Bates, Larry Fenson, David Taylor, Daphne Maurer, Terri Lewis, Larry Weiskrantz, Tony Moore, Faraneh Vargha-Khadem, Lily and Victor Dubowitz, Francis Cowan, John Wyatt, Stuart Judge, Mary Rutherford, Judith Meek, Graeme Bydder, Lynn Murray, Semir Zeki, John Stein, Patrick Cavanagh, Giovanni Cioni and Anna Chilosi, Tim Shallice and Maria Tallandini, Johannes Zanker, Bob Turner, Alastair Fielder, Patricia Sonksen, Richard Frackowiak, Annette Karmiloff-Smith, Orlee Udwin, and Uta Frith.

The theme of this book is to trace over the past 20 years the growth of our understanding of brain structure–function relationships in visual development. There is no attempt to be completely comprehensive, but rather to pick out the landmark experiments and point out the present gaps in knowledge (which are huge in some areas). I concentrate on early visual development over the first 2 years of life, but some of the changes discussed continue for many years and so are discussed up to adult maturity.

In Chapter 1, there is a brief history of the field, emphasizing my own neuroscientific approach and contrasting it with others that are perhaps considered more psychological or medical.

Research on visual development is a very practical, hands-on area of research with much of the research being driven by invention of new techniques and measures. In Chapter 2 there is an account of current methods used to measure visual development. Some of these methods have been pioneered in our own laboratory and have been important steps in the progress of the VDU's research.

In Chapter 3 the main theoretical framework is outlined. I start from the original theory of two visual systems—a division between a phylogenetically old and new—subcortical and cortical. This idea formed the basis for all our early work. This natural division has perhaps become less distinct over the past 20 years, as we become more aware of different functionally separate cortical and subcortical streams and modules and the very complex interactions between them in development. Here the theory of development of vision takes off from adult and animal research, but has a number of interesting twists when considering human infants. The next theoretical change has been to move full circle back to a largely Piagetian idea of visual development, where change is driven by new strategies for actions, rather than as a result of passive perceptual processing. Taking the theoretical stance of Goodale and Milner, with the division of the cortex into the ventral visual stream (for perception) and dorsal visual stream (for action) we can start to redefine developmental 'visuomotor action modules' and perceptual 'object recognition modules' within the infant's brain. The final development of the theory must be to consider integration of information across visual streams with the development of executive decision-making skills in the child. Traditionally, this has been seen as 'cognitive development' but I will make the claim that from a neurobiological prospective the dividing lines between perception and cognition are somewhat blurred.

In Chapters 4–7 the development of various brain modules underlying different visual attributes is discussed. We will start in Chapter 4 with the newborn's vision, with measures of acuity and contrast sensitivity, which are usually taken as the milestones of early visual development. When discussing limiting factors in acuity we need to take into account changes in the optical properties of the growing eye. Using some of the new techniques we have developed we have run two major vision screening programmes, specifically for understanding the optical focusing abilities which change with age and the relationship between these and amblyopia and strabismus. A whole book could be dedicated to discussion of this topic alone, but in Chapter 5 we outline what is understood at present about refractive changes in development and links to development of accommodation and stereopsis. Specific cortical modules for orientation, disparity detection, relative motion, and relative pattern parameters are discussed in Chapter 6. In Chapter 7 visual ventral stream functioning for object and face perception is briefly discussed. In Chapter 8 we discuss our current knowledge of development of 'action streams' and their relationship to developing selective attention. The two main action modules we have researched are those of eye movement control, related to attention and hand–eye movement systems. Two very important later - developing action systems, locomotion and speech, will not be covered as they are beyond the scope of this book.

Speech and locomotion have not been the focus of the VDU's research, although we have recently adapted the MacArthur Communication Inventory (devised by Liz Bates, Larry Fenson, and their colleagues) from American English to UK English and have started to look at the development of walking and its integration with space perception mechanisms. A remaining question is why we get sequential development of these various action systems and what triggers the next action system to become functional and eventually mature. An intriguing possibility is that limitations in both visual attentional systems and those underlying spatial representation limit the functioning of action systems at different stages of development. I am afraid that we have very incomplete answers in many of these areas, but the hope is that this discussion will introduce the reader to a much broader interdisciplinary approach to visual development than is currently often taken, and perhaps trigger research enthusiasm for those starting in this type of work.

Much of our work over the past years has been motivated by attempting to find better ways to diagnose early visual problems and to devise ways of combating visual disability. In assessing vision in infants and children with a wide range of clinical problems, from those at the more sensory and peripheral end, e.g. cataract and glaucoma, to those with more central neural systems affected, e.g. those with perinatal brain damage, Williams syndrome, and visual dyslexia, we are always trying to add to our theoretical understanding of plasticity within development. Throughout this book I will use examples from our clinical findings to discuss the plasticity of specific eye–brain modules. However, these ideas will be summarized in Chapter 9, where I consider plasticity at different levels of the visual system. The conclusion from our research to date is that many of the developmental abnormalities we consider are due to relative dorsal stream vulnerability compared with ventral stream vulnerability.

In Chapter 10 I attempt to outline questions for the future both in basic and clinical research and emphasize the value of multidisciplinary research teams, tackling research problems at different levels of analysis in parallel.

This preface ends with first, an apology to any readers who feel offended that their particular contribution to our understanding of developing vision has been left out. As I have been writing I am aware that I am losing the battle to be completely up-to-date, and have not got the space to consider all the areas I think should be included under visual development. I am also acutely aware of lacunae in my own knowledge, but hope you will enjoy reading this book and forgive my omissions.

Secondly, you will find that when you read this book I sometimes refer to 'our studies' or 'our model' or 'we have found' rather than using the first person singular or the passive third person. This is because infant research cannot be carried out by one person alone, it depends on a co-ordinated team, with different members contributing to different aspects of the study. It is not the royal 'we' which I use, but an indication of the collaborative nature of all my research.

Thirdly, I would like to thank all the staff of Oxford University Press, and in particular Vanessa Whiting for her extreme patience in waiting for me to finish this book. I am afraid that the major move to UCL with the setting up and running of two groups in London and Cambridge, plus our involvement in UCL academically have all added to the delay, but also provided us with lots of new thoughts and experiences about infant development.

Finally I would like to thank my family for all their support. Besides Ol there are my mother and sister, Sue; my children—Fleur, Hugo, Lorrin, and Ione; my niece, Zoe; and Ol's mother, Midge. They have helped me see things in perspective and understand better the symbiosis between one's life as a researcher and one's life as a member of a family. Most importantly, I thank Ol Braddick. I have always wished I could clone him in that he has so many diverse competences and abilities inside one set of genes. His intellectual capacities to debate and discuss scientific issues at many different levels and to extract the core message, has always been an inspiration to me. This book is really the joint work of two life-long collaborators and would not have been finished without Ol's help at the more practical level of sorting out and finding references, drawing figures, taking photographs, correcting grammar and spelling in the text, and most of all, supporting and loving me over many years.

J. Atkinson

Contents

Glossary

fMRI	functional magnetic resonance imaging
FPL	forced-choice preferential looking
HIE	hypoxic–ischaemic encephalopathy
IOR	inhibition of return
LGN	lateral geniculate nucleus
MOKN	monocular optokinetic nystagmus
NMDA	N-methyl-D-aspartate
OKN	optokinetic nystagmus
OR VEP	orientation reversal visual evoked potential
PL	preferential looking
VEP	visual evoked potential
VERP	visual event related potential

1 Background context

1.1 MAJOR INFLUENCES

The research and ideas in this book have been largely influenced by the neuroscientific approach to both adult visual psychophysics and electrophysiological and anatomical studies on other species. However, other approaches to the development of vision, by those coming from perceptual and cognitive psychology and from paediatric neurology and ophthalmology have also influenced our ideas and theories. These background influences are briefly discussed here, but detailed reviews can be found elsewhere.

1.2 INFLUENCES FROM ADULT AND ANIMAL NEUROSCIENCE

There are two major neuroscientific research methodologies which influenced our early research in visual development. One is the pioneering work in electrophysiology by such giants as Hubel and Wiesel, Mountcastle, and Barlow; for the first time the activity in individual cells in the brain was linked to the detection of particular visual attributes, elucidating bottom-up hierarchical subsystems. These were the first serious attempts to link anatomical structure to brain function in vision.

Together with these findings came the idea of the development of the visual system being modifiable within a 'critical period' by environmental forces in the form of particular types of visual stimulation and deprivation. One of the first important results was that of Wiesel and Hubel (1963) on neurons in the primary visual cortex of a cat. They found that these neurons were normally capable of being activated by stimulation of either eye, but lost the input from one eye if that eye was deprived of vision early in life. However, if both eyes are deprived of vision early in life, it seems that the neurons remain sensitive to inputs from both eyes. This led to the idea of cortical competition, where the sensitivity of cells in the developing cortex are dependent on the parameters of the early visual environment. Of course, clinically it had been known for over a century that, if vision was prevented early in life because of an occluding cataract or a deviating eye in strabismus, removal of the cataract, or surgery to straighten the eyes, rarely resulted in any useful vision in the operated eye. However, the electrophysiological results started to lead to an understanding of the underlying mechanism, elucidating the brain areas which were critical for normal visual development. Extensive studies of critical periods in cat and monkey vision followed in the seventies, led by Colin Blakemore, Jack Pettigrew, Nigel Daw, Don Mitchell, and their colleagues and research students.

The other important influence from neuroscience at the time was the theory put forward by Fergus Campbell and John Robson (1968), who suggested that the brain contained populations or streams of neurons, tuned to different spatial frequencies, which operated in an analogous fashion to linear Fourier analysis. They revealed the existence of spatial frequency channels by using adaptation and masking paradigms. Much of our early experimental work on infants was based on modifying these adult psychophysical methods to compare infant development with adult capabilities.

Extensive neuroanatomical and physiological studies in the seventies and early eighties enabled theorists to use these results to hypothesize division of the adult visual system into functional subsystems (or channels, streams or modules). Each module may be involved with processing particular types of visual information—for example, there is a cortical module specifically designed to analyse the contrasting wavelengths or colour of objects. The ideas of these channels was not entirely new— Kenneth Craik (1966), a remarkable experimental psychologist working in the Applied Psychology Unit in Cambridge, had already theorized along these lines much earlier and the information theorists, using ideas from communication engineers, had already analysed visual arrays in terms of specific limited capacity channels. Donald Broadbent's influential 'filter' theory of cognition (Broadbent, 1958) in which he hypothesized a selective filter which can be tuned to any of a large number of channels for perceptual information, used the Craik channel theory as a starting point. The specialized filters idea is also the basis of current influential theories such as the *working memory* model of Alan Baddeley (Baddeley and Hitch, 1974).

Having started off in infant vision researching the basic visual attributes of acuity, contrast sensitivity, and binocularity, we began to hypothesize about the development of different brain subsystems or channels and the interactions between them. From about the mid-seventies there has been one simple predominant idea which formed the basis of all our theorizing on early visual development in the first year of life. This is based on the idea of two distinct visual systems—a subcortical one and a cortical one. The subcortical system controls all reflex eye movements in orienting, while the cortical system controls shifts of visual attention, understanding, visual recognition, and memory. In fact all the processes that are included in 'visual perception and cognition'—the analysis, categorization, and understanding of incoming visual sensory information, combined with linking this information to communicative systems and motor actions—involve cortical functioning. The exploration of these cortical channels forms the basis for much of the research reported in this book.

All the neurobiological experimentation and theories of vision mentioned above assume that certain visual areas and pathways between the eye and brain are thought to 'mature', due to an interaction between genetically prewired programming and environmentally dependent learning. These changes produce measurable parallel behavioural changes. Many assumptions, some quite questionable, are made about the 1 : 1 relationship between physiological changes and the observed changes in behaviour. Of course, the act of identifying the maturation of a particular part of the eye–brain system, which is paralleled by a specific change in visual capacity or behaviour, should never be regarded as a complete understanding of the developmental processes underlying change. A yet more abstract level of analysis would specify the relationship between a change in visual behaviour and the development of thought processes (or level of conscious understanding) underlying this change. In some respects the more 'psychological' approaches to visual development have attempted to analyse development at these more abstract levels.

1.3 INFLUENCES FROM PERCEPTUAL AND COGNITIVE PSYCHOLOGY

The 'psychological' theories tend not to use the neuroanatomical or physiological data but rather they consider visual development as divided into different stages or levels of processing. Each level of processing represents a different level of cognitive understanding. Some theorists think of these different levels of understanding as different types of representation. As the child develops, more elaborate levels of cognitive analysis are seen as the child's understanding shifts from a relatively naive theory to more complex adult-like levels of representation and integration.

The starting point of psychological theorizing on development is encapsulated in the theorizing of Piaget. Piaget (1953) assumed that information from the different senses, including vision, gradually becomes co-ordinated through active experience and learning. He thought of observed behaviour as being divided into distinct schemas (each schema being a co-ordinated set of motor acts). Piaget hypothesized that perceptuocognitive development takes place through two internal processes, *assimilation* and *accommodation*. In *assimilation* new sensory events are incorporated into existing schemas, whereas in *accommodation* entirely new schemas are formed because new experiences cannot be incorporated into existing ones. Piaget's view assumed that the perceptual capacities of the infant in the first 6 months were very limited. This was largely because the tasks he devised to test perceptual understanding depended very heavily on competent motor control of the body, arm, and hand, which the infant clearly did not have early in life. However, his emphasis on *active* learning and his detailed descriptions of infant behaviour led the way for developmentalists to extend Piagetian ideas back to early infancy, considering the more mature eye movement systems, rather than immature eye–hand movement systems, as the basis for development of schemas in early life.

Gibson (1950) in his theorizing held almost the opposite view to Piaget. He argued that sensation and perception were a single process of seeking out information and that 'seeing' depended on radiant transmission of the patterned light reflected from the texture or pattern on objects and surfaces. He hypothesized that the newborn infant already possessed mature 'higher-order structures', such as mechanisms for analysing texture gradients (the change in retinal size of texture elements dependent on viewing distance) which carry information for direct analysis. According to Gibson, newborns can perceive the real shape and size of objects effortlessly and can innately relate information from different senses. Complex perceptual understanding of spatial relations is available to the infant because they can organize incoming sensory information effortlessly and automatically in an adult-like fashion. There have been extensive attempts, in particular by Tom Bower (1974) and Liz Spelke (Spelke *et al.*, 1992; Spelke, 1994) to demonstrate innate automatic adult-like perception and cognition, as evidence of complex representations, already present in newborns. For example, Bower has claimed that young infants change their visual expression to one representing 'surprise' (to an adult) if a toy, which has previously been visibly hidden behind a screen, is not visible when the screen is removed ('invisible disappearance'). For Bower the infant's brain must contain working processes which store visual memories of the toy over time and functional mechanisms to understand that solid objects like toys are not destroyed by the screen, but go on existing behind the screen when hidden. There must also be links within the infant's brain to register these insights by means of a change in visual expression, which can be universally recognized as expressing a particular emotion by other human beings. Others have demonstrated similar complex levels of understanding of object permanence in relatively young infants. For example, 4-month-old infants have been shown to look longer at a display which still contains two objects when they have previously seen one object already removed from the two-object display. Karen Wynn argues that this shows some rudimentary understanding or recognition of addition and subtraction (Wynn 1992). These debates concerning complex representations that seem to be operating at birth will be returned to, when newborn capacities are discussed in Chapter 4.

1.4 NATURE–NURTURE

The nature–nurture debate over what exactly is already specified in the genetic prewiring and what is modified through experience has occurred over and over again in visual development both within the neuroscientific approach and in more traditional developmental psychological theorizing. Most theorists accept that adult visual capacities are the result of complex interactions between genes and environment, but the nature of this interaction is often incompletely specified. These interactions can be considered at different levels. Some of these interactions are at the molecular and cellular level whereas others are discussed at a level between the child and the external environment. For some aspects of visual development it may be useful to distinguish between environmental factors which are typical for the species and factors which are specific to the individual. Mark Johnson and John Morton (Morton and Johnson 1991) have used this distinction between prototype face perception and recognition of individual faces in their theory of face perception in infancy. This will be considered further in Chapter 4.

Much of our current understanding of genetic–environmental interactions in human visual development come from detailed studies of the effects of environmental manipulation on changes in visual brain processing in the cat and monkey (for an excellent review of this literature see Daw 1995). The pioneering work of Hubel and Wiesel, discussed above, demonstrated the necessity of registered binocular pattern stimulation for development of normal binocular vision and analogies were made between the changes in binocular cortex seen in the animal brain and the infant brain suffering from congenital strabismus (cross eyes).

As well as considering the level of these interactions, it is very important to consider the timing of them. In visual development this debate has centred around the idea of 'critical' or 'sensitive' time periods. A critical period is defined as the period of time when the course of visual development can be modified by changes in the visual input. It is known that, in general, all development is considered to be more modifiable early in life than in adulthood, and this has been believed to be true for human visual development for many years. However, it is now clear that there are many different critical periods for different parts of visual processing, and that there may also be individual differences in plasticity within different systems. Nigel Daw has put forward a general rule which is that plasticity persists at higher levels of the system for longer than at lower levels of the system so, for example, the critical period for ocular dominance changes end later in output layers than in input layers. This means that the critical period in the cat for orientation and direction, which is created by activity in input layers of visual cortex, has virtually ended at 6 weeks of age while the critical period for development of ocular dominance changes extends well beyond this period because it is dependent on changes in both input and output layers (Daw and Wyatt 1976). There appears to be a longer time period of plasticity the more complex the visual processing, so although the retina is largely hard-wired at birth the visual cortex appears to be plastic early in life, with areas of the temporal cortex and hippocampus remaining plastic up until adulthood and possibly throughout life.

Consideration of critical periods and the plasticity of different visual processing modules will be reconsidered in Chapter 9; for example, the extra visual experience of premature babies and the abnormal visual input of children with eye defects such as cataract and strabismus.

1.5 NEWER INFLUENCES FROM NEURAL IMAGING

We can now add data from new methods of neuroimaging, where functional maps of brain activity are produced based on metabolic changes in blood flow or electrical activity. Examples of these are positron emission tomography and functional magnetic resonance imaging (fMRI). Both at present have a number of difficulties with their use in young infants, but we are already able to use analogies from adult studies for understanding the infant brain. Hopefully, in the next few years, it will be possible to use modifications of these techniques to gain insights into the developing brain in human infants.

1.6 CONCLUSIONS

Although much of our research has relied heavily on the neurophysiological results from other species combined, more recently, with results from fMRI studies on adults, our ideas have been tempered by the approaches of developmental psychology and the results of clinical research on patient populations both in paediatric neurology and ophthalmology. No single approach can give us an understanding of visual development at all levels of analysis, and although there may be gaps between the results from different approaches at present, our theoretical accounts are moving towards a synthesis of these approaches.

Chapter 2 looks in more detail at the methodologies which have been used combining these approaches, before moving on to the theoretical accounts in Chapter 3.

2 Paediatric vision testing

Measuring visual abilities in infants and young children is a skill which requires not only careful design of the test material, but also scientific and social skills, to take into account the practical and ethical limitations of working with babies and young children. One obvious limitation is that, unlike adults, infants cannot follow verbal instructions and cannot deliver verbal responses. Toddlers and pre-school children may be able to give you a verbal answer, but they may not have understood the question in the same way as an adult. In addition, 3–6 year olds find it extremely hard to 'guess', especially if a stimulus is near their visual threshold. Near threshold they often refuse to go on or show strong biases. There is not usually the possibility of exposing infants to controlled stimulus contingencies over an extended period of time, and the motivational manipulations that help to establish learning in animals are not usually ethically or practically possible. Consequently, a set of electrophysiological and behavioural psychophysical methods has been developed and adapted which are appropriate for the limited range of behaviour in the child's normal repertoire. This behavioural repertoire varies widely with age (and mental age for clinical groups), making the analysis of individual changes in vision, measured longitudinally, quite complex. It is often necessary to use different methods for different ages, and this can complicate the interpretation of changes in development with age.

In addition, infants and children vary in mood or 'state' quite rapidly over time. Various scales have been devised to gauge 'state' at the time of testing. For example, Heinz Prechtl (1974) has devised a five-point scale, indicating changes of state in infants. At one end of the scale there is 'deep sleep', while at the other end there is 'awake and actively crying'. Somewhere in the middle is state 3—'awake, alert and calm', the ideal state for testing infants. In general the easier the task and more varied the stimuli the longer an infant or young child will co-operate. But in newborns changes of state across the five-point scale can vary over a few minutes. This usually means that to engage a newborn infant in a visual experiment will require the testing to last not more than 5–10 min. Toddlers, rather than crying or dropping asleep as is the case in newborns, get bored very quickly and opt out of the testing situation. Two to 3 year olds have very definite ideas about what they want to do at any moment and so you will notice that the number of publications on this age group are very few!

One limiting factor in measuring infants' visual capacities is the ability of the child's motor system in controlling eye and limb movements and in general support of the body and head. The newborn (which can be defined as the first postnatal month in term infants) has some control over head and eye movements and so fixation behaviour can be used as a behavioural indicator. Between birth and 6 months, infants show an increasing readiness to shift fixation briskly and accurately between targets in the field of view; the fastest saccade are essentially adult-like, although there is likely to be more variability than in the adult. Many of the successful behavioural studies of infant vision, throughout the first year of life, have depended on fixation behaviour. However, in assessing abnormal vision it is often difficult to separate poor eye and head movement control from more central cognitive deficits.

For older infants and toddlers, motoric limitations in reaching, grasping, and walking are also important to take into account. There is some evidence that whole arm movements may be crudely directed by the newborn towards targets of interest, but in general these responses are not sufficiently reliable to be a useful response measure in vision testing of individual infants. From about 4 months onwards, infants start to make visually directed arm movements; initially, these reach a target in a number of corrective steps, but over the period between 4 and 18 months an increasing proportion of reaches occur in a single, smooth ballistic action. From 6 to 12 months the behaviour of reaching for a small visually presented object can appear quite compulsive, although rather little is known about the visual properties that determine this behaviour.

Infants require considerable postural support for any of these behaviours to be studied. Some researchers studying infants in the first 2 months of life have presented visual displays above the infant, with the child in a supine position. This may make access for comforting or adjusting the infant's position difficult, and there is also a concern that young infants are more likely to go into a drowsy state when lying down. For these reasons, most studies have involved testing infants in a seated posture. There are many alternatives here from a human 'holder' to a specially moulded chair for the individual baby. I have tried many of these at one time or another with different ages and different tests, but have come to the conclusion that with babies under 6 months the best results are with infants sitting semi-upright on a supportive adult and for over 6 months usually this adult has to be a familiar caregiver to prevent the child becoming distressed by strangers. There is concern that the holder may try to aid the responses of the infant (particularly if the holder is the parent) during testing; however, on informal testing, where even if you deliberately try, as the holder, to turn the infant's body and direct the eyes to a particular location, this is usually impossible to do. Most infants show very definite looking patterns decided by themselves, not the holder or tester.

Infant vision research depends on working with vulnerable subjects who cannot themselves give consent to test procedures. They are in the test unit with the consent of their parents who are concerned to protect their child from any risk or discomfort. Ethically, it is essential that not only are there no objective risks to the child, but also that parents are entirely confident that their baby is happy and comfortable, and that they fully understand what is going on. For the success of research in infant vision, the interpersonal skills of the tester are as significant as skill in display calibration or data analysis. All of the research of the Visual Development Unit has depended on the interpersonal skills and team co-operation of members of the group and none of the research from the group would have been possible without the multiple skills of all concerned.

2.1 BEHAVIOURAL AND ELECTROPHYSIOLOGICAL METHODS FOR INFANT TESTING

2.1.1 Infant eye movements

As much of the knowledge about the development of human vision rests on evidence from eye movements, this section will start with a brief overview of their development (good examples of reviews on infant eye movements are by Hainline 1993 and by Shupert and Fuchs 1988).

Saccadic dynamics seem to be essentially adult-like at an early age (Hainline *et al*. 1984; Hainline 1993), although at 1 month saccades have been reported to be hypotonic, i.e. fall short of their targets under some stimulus conditions (e.g. Aslin and Salapatek 1975). The ease with which competing stimuli can elicit a saccade, and the latency with which they do so, change markedly with age and are revealing about the development of systems for the control of visual attention.

For most test situations with discrete targets there are only very brief episodes of smooth pursuit before about 2 months of age (e.g. Aslin 1981; Hainline 1985, 1993). However, some researchers have reported small episodes of smooth pursuit for very low velocities of target movement in newborns. In contrast, optokinetic nystagmus (OKN) elicited by large-field motion is present from birth and if the smooth pursuit part of the OKN cycle is considered to be the same in terms of dynamics as smooth pursuit eye movements made to follow a single target, then it must be accepted that the kinetic mechanisms of smooth pursuit are fairly mature at birth. An initial OKN asymmetry (called 'MOKN' for monocular OKN), for the first months of life has been found when monocular rather than binocular stimulation is used (Atkinson and Braddick 1981*b*). Interpretation of the change-over from asymmetrical MOKN to symmetrical responses will be considered in Chapter 6.

The development of vergence movements of the eyes (where the two eyes move towards or away from each other) is important for understanding the development of binocularity. A substantial degree of vergence control appears to be present before the onset of sensitivity to binocular correlation and disparity at about 10–16 weeks of age (Aslin 1993; Hainline and Riddell 1996) raising the unanswered question as to what drives infant vergence, if not disparity. There has been considerable debate about the alignment of the two eyes in newborn infants. As newborns have a larger angle kappa than adults (the angle between the optic and visual axes of the eye), when one studies alignment by measuring corneal reflectance in each eye, many experimenters have found that newborn infants appear divergent. This may often be an artefactual result due to their enlarged angle kappa.

2.1.2 Measuring eye movements

Almost all preferential-looking and habituation-recovery experiments depend on an observer judging the infant's direction of gaze, either directly or by video observation. Fortunately, a human observer is highly sensitive to another's gaze direction, especially with respect to a straight-ahead position (so it is important that the observation position should be centred with respect to the display). The minimum size of eye and head movement to be reliably judged is about 5 degrees visual angle. The judgement is greatly aided by observing the reflection of the stimulus in the cornea. For video observation, this can be enhanced by positioning infra-red light-emitting diodes symmetrically with respect to the display or within the video camera.

Direct observation yields information on fixations that is quite adequate for preference and habituation studies, but it can tell us little about the quantitative precision, timing, or kinematics of eye movements. Examination of a videotaped record can give information about the onset time and duration of movements (if the 50/60 Hz time resolution of standard video is adequate), although the analysis is tedious, especially if the movements of interest have to be found by searching the taped records. We have used this method for looking at the development of attention in infants and in looking at eye movements during OKN (see studies in Chapter 6 and 9).

2.2 COMMON METHODS USED IN STUDYING DEVELOPING VISION—FROM INFANCY TO SCHOOL AGE

2.2.1 Preferential looking

Preferential looking is the most widely used method for testing infants' ability to make visual discriminations. It is based on the logic that an infant who shows a sta-

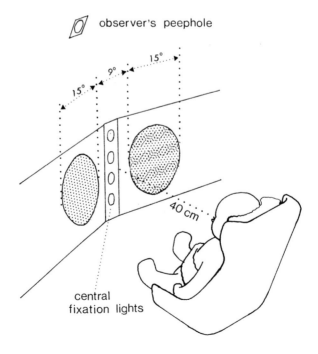

Fig. 2.1(a)

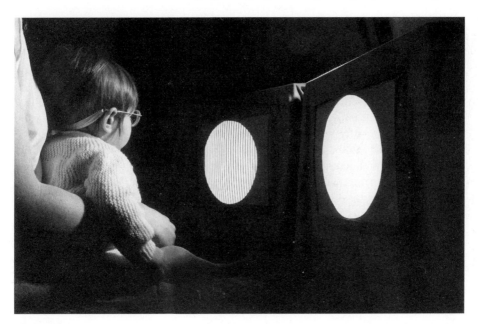

Fig. 2.1(b)

Fig. 2.1 (a) A schematic of the forced-choice preferential looking set-up. (b) Photograph taken in the forced-choice preferential looking apparatus.

tistically reliable preference for stimulus A (the 'positive stimulus') over stimulus B (the 'negative stimulus' or 'foil') must be able to discriminate between A and B. In particular, infants have a preference for looking at a patterned field rather than a homogeneous field, which has been used extensively to assess acuity or contrast sensitivity. The method was introduced by Fantz (e.g. Fantz *et al.* 1962), but most modern work has used the version known as *forced-choice preferential looking* (FPL), introduced by Davida Teller for measuring visual acuity.

Figure 2.1 shows a schematic of the PL set-up, and the FPL automated apparatus, used in our unit's baby lab. Stimuli are displayed at two locations at the child's eye level and either side of the midline. On each trial, one side displays the positive (patterned) stimulus, and the other a uniform field matched in mean luminance. The observer views the child's face either directly through a peephole or via a video camera, from a midline location. The observer does not know which is the positive side on each trial (this is randomly selected either by a computer controlling the stimulus, or by a second tester). The observer has to make a 'blind' decision (a 'forced choice') as to which side the infant preferred on each trial. The observer can use any behaviour of the infant to help decision making: eye movements, head movements, state or mood changes, whole body movements, and so on. The observation period is under the observer's control and does not usually exceed 10 s. Psychophysical staircase procedures have usually been used in studies in our own Unit, and more details of the methodology can be found elsewhere (see for example, Atkinson and Braddick 1998).

The FPL procedure has been extended to test for a preference between two patterned fields, one of which contains some feature or large-scale organization lacking in the other. Examples of these will be given in Chapter 6. In at least some cases, the preference between two patterns is clearly less marked than in acuity testing, presumably because even the 'negative stimulus' contains enough detail and contrast to be attractive to the child. Compared with acuity testing, the observer may well be required to observe a longer sample of fixation behaviour before reaching a decision on each trial. Recently, PL has been used where the choice is between two solid objects or virtual 3D shapes on a computer screen and these preferences have been compared with 'preferential reaching', measuring reaching preferences (which objects is touched and manipulated), between pairs of solid objects. These studies will be referred to in Chapter 8.

2.2.2 Teller/Keeler cards

Display of the grating patterns on cards rather than electronically have been produced by Davida Teller and Alistair Fielder's groups (e.g. McDonald *et al.* 1985). Acuity cards, commercially available as the Teller Acuity Cards or the Keeler Acuity Cards, are an adaptation of the PL procedure for the estimation of infants' acuity in clinical settings. A grating is printed in one window on one side of a card, with the rest of the card matching grey. Alternatively, there may be a patch of grey pattern on the opposite side to the stripes, the patch being matched in size and mean luminance to the striped patch. Each card is held up by the observer, who views the infant through a central peephole. The observer, who can choose to present the card either way or both ways round, has to judge whether the infant prefers to look at one side or the other. Reliability of the acuity estimates within about 1 octave has been demonstrated (Mash *et al.* 1995). However, this is not often a forced-choice procedure, as it is not necessarily carried out 'blind' on the part of the observer. In many clinical settings one tester will arrange the order of the cards and know the side of grating on presentation.

2.2.3 Acuity measures beyond infancy

It is sometimes difficult to sustain interest long enough, even with a short staircase procedure, to get a reliable PL acuity measure from a child aged over 12–18 months. Some results in older children have been obtained with an operant variant, where fixating the patterned stimulus is rewarded by the appearance of an animated toy (e.g. Mayer and Dobson 1980). Contrast sensitivity has been measured successfully in 10 month olds using an operant procedure in which the infant was auditorily reinforced with a tinkling bell for picking up the striped rattle (covered in a grating pattern) rather than the rattle covered in plain grey, matched in mean luminance to the stripes (Atkinson and French 1983) (see Fig. 2.2). However, many of these operant procedures take longer to run than PL making them unlikely to yield more reliable results, particularly with clinical populations where an individual infant's results are important rather than collecting age-group average data.

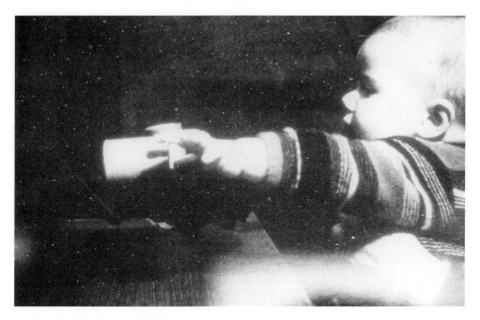

Fig. 2.2 Operant procedure for measuring contrast sensitivity in infants. The cylinder covered in stripes is auditory reinforcing when lifted by the child (it contains a tinkling bell).

From about $3\frac{1}{2}$ years, children can usually understand the demands of a simple matching task, so that optotypes of graded sizes or pictures of objects can be used as stimuli without the need for the child 'naming' the object. Single optotypes, such as the STYCAR letters (Sheridan 1976) are known to overestimate acuity relative to arrangements of letters in adult letter naming charts (e.g. Snellen, Bailey-Lovie) . In these adult charts there are possible 'crowding' interactions between the letters. Because these adult letter naming charts are not practical with most 3–6 year olds, we developed a test for measuring 'crowded' acuity, calling it the Cambridge Crowding Cards (see Fig. 2.3).

Here the child is asked to match only the central letter from a cross-shaped array of five letters (Atkinson *et al.* 1986*a*, 1988*a*). Such tests have proved particularly useful in the study of amblyopia and will be returned to in Chapter 9. It has also been found that many developmental dyslexics show marked crowding on the Cambridge Crowding Cards, but only when each eye is tested separately in monocular viewing (Atkinson 1993). In monocular viewing the disparity cue to focus is abolished and without this the task seems to require more attention, so it seems possible that a relationship between focusing, disparity, and attentional factors may be the explanation for this result in dyslexics.

A rather similar test to the Cambridge Crowding Cards, but using a linear optotype display, has been developed by Patricia Sonksen and Janet Silver (Sonsken and Silver 1988; Salt *et al.* 1995), called the Sonksen–Silver Cards. We initially compared,

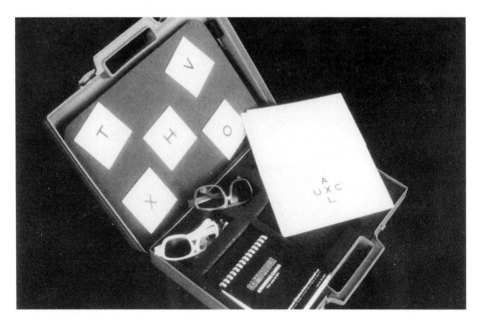

Fig 2.3 Cambridge Crowding Cards and matching board. The size of letters is varied across cards, but the ratio of letter size to spacing of the letters is kept constant. The child has a matching board and has to point on their board to the central letter on the card. The child views the crowded card at a distance of 3 m.

the ease of use of linear displays with the circular or cross shaped array, and found that for 4–6 year olds there was more variability in using the linear array, because the child often became confused as to which particular letter in the array was the one to be matched (Atkinson *et al.* 1986*a*). Consequently, it was decided to use only the cross-shaped array in the final version of the Cambridge Crowding Cards.

We have also used boxes or surrounding lines around letters to be identified rather than surrounding letters (Atkinson 1991). Surrounding lines can also produce a 'crowding' effect (similar in extent to the surrounding letters in adults). In young children the surrounding letters seem to require additional skills of selective attention compared with surrounding lines and so can give a reduced value of visual acuity in children with attentional deficits.

2.2.4 Habituation methods

The visual habituation measure is based on the simple observation that infants fixate objects and people around them and once they are familiar with them they show a decrement in looking at the familiar stimulus. This decrement in attention is called 'habituation' and represents a measure of a primitive form of learning. This waxing and waning of visual attention has been seen in many laboratory settings but is also observed in naturalistic environments such as infants attending to faces and objects encountered at home (e.g. Bornstein and Ludemann 1989). A number of studies have shown that habituation is similar in infants from different cultures (e.g. Bornstein *et al*. 1988) and to be a reasonably reliable measure for an individual infant over short periods of time (e.g. Bornstein and Benasich 1986; Mayes and Kessen 1989).

It has been used widely in measuring visual development of attentional processes and for visual discriminations ranging from spatial phase discrimination to colour categorization and face discrimination. When it is used for measuring discriminations the infant becomes habituated by repeated exposure to a stimulus A, thus enhancing a novelty preference for a second stimulus B, which is shown to the infant after habituation to A. A visual preference for B then provides evidence that the infants can discriminate between A and B.

In practice, habituation can be quantified by a variety of measures—length of first look, the longest look, the looking times over a certain number of looks, or the cumulative time before the habituation criterion is reached. Some infants decrease their looking times monotonically from their first look, others first increase their looking times over the first few looks and then decrease or fluctuate. In general, habituation occurs more rapidly the older the infant, but varies across individual infants within one age group. There have been many variants of the basic habituation procedure (Bornstein 1985). However, to meet the requirement that habituation has occurred to a common level across individuals, a modification called the 'infant-control' procedure is used (after Horowitz *et al*. 1972). A typical procedure used is shown in Fig. 2.4.

The use of simultaneous presentation in the test phase has been found by us and others to be more sensitive than successive presentation in some cases (Slater *et al*. 1988; Atkinson *et al*. 1988*b*).

In some experiments, it is not possible to confine differences between the habituated and novel stimuli to the variable that the experimenter wishes to investigate. For example, in investigating infants' sensitivity to phase relations in compound gratings, the desired question is whether an infant, habituated to one particular phase relationship, responds to the novelty of another phase relationship regardless of variations in peak to trough contrast in the grating stimulus. Unfortunately, discrimination in this case could rest on merely the contrast of the grating, as it is known that in general infants prefer to look at high contrast rather than low contrast gratings, if the spatial frequency is above acuity threshold. This problem can be resolved by varying the habituation stimulus in a dimension which is irrelevant to the discrimination. For example, in a study on relative phase discrimination (Braddick *et al*. 1986*b*), the overall peak to trough contrast was varied from trial to trial in the habituation phase but the relative phase was kept constant. This ensures that infants' responses to the novelty of a stimulus with different spatial phase relations was not based on the difference in peak-to-trough contrast, but was based on the spatial configuration.

Habituation/dishabituation procedures have been used by many developmental psychologists to investigate a wide variety of the infant's perceptual and cognitive visual understanding. For example, Spelke and Van de Walle (1993) have used the habituation procedure to study how infants perceive the unity of objects as a whole, distinct from their surroundings. Bertenthal *et al*. (1984) have used the method to

---

HABITUATION PHASE

Habituation trials
- Infant turned towards screen; when fixating centrally, habituation pattern is turned on.
- Observer holds down button for time infant fixates pattern.
- When infant has looked away for 2 s, pattern display automatically terminated. Infant is then turned away.
- Looking time over each set of three consecutive trials automatically totalled.
- Habituation criterion reached when three-trial total has fallen to 50% or less of its maximum value.

TEST PHASE

Test trials – sequential
- Four successive trials, alternating 'novel' and habituation' pattern; counterbalanced across infants.
- Timing procedures as in habituation phase.

Test trials – simultaneous
- Two trials with 'novel' and 'habituation' patterns displayed side by side, one on either side of the midline, counterbalanced for side of pattern on first trial and second trial (to cancel out effects of any side bias).
- The observer records, on two buttons, the duration of fixations to each pattern.
- Trial is automatically terminated when total looking time for the two stimuli reaches 20 s.

Fig. 2.4 Habituation procedure.

show that 3 and 5 month olds show sensitivity to biological motion in point light displays (the lights being attached to the major joints of a walking figure, with the figure being invisible except for the lights). Bornstein (1998) reviews evidence that early measures of habituation in individual infants can be related to indicators of intelligence in later childhood.

However, there are still unanswered fundamental questions concerning the underlying mechanisms which cause habituation. Habituation taken simply as a reduced responsiveness with familiarity, has been demonstrated from single organisms throughout the animal kingdom, and does not require highly evolved nervous systems to demonstrate the phenomena. However, successful habituation does imply some minimal neurological integration of sensory incoming information with perceptual encoding and memory processing. In our infant studies we have often considered it a shorthand for 'short-term attentional salience', building in the assumption that the infant is capable of linking the interest value of a stimulus with its looking time. As such, habituation has been considered to reflect the construction of some sort of internal representation, with this representation being continuously compared with the stimulus that is presently on view. Sokolov (1963) in his 'comparator model' assumed that the decline in attention in habituation was directly related to the efficiency with which the organism forms a representation of the stimulus. If incoming information about the stimulus matches the representation, then the organism will not go on attending to the stimulus because there is no new information to be gained from doing so. However, if there is a mismatch, then attention to the external stimulus will be continued, as is the case with the novel stimulus in the post-habituation phase. This view of habituation equates the mechanism with selection, encoding, and retention of information from the environment.

It is reasonable to suppose from this that infants who process more efficiently, should acquire knowledge of the stimulus more quickly and stop looking at it sooner. This should be reflected in shorter peak durations and accumulated looking times, and quicker decays; assuming that this reflects rapid production of the central representation and comparison. Weight has been given to these arguments from the adult literature where a strong correlation has been found between inspection time and intelligence test performance (e.g. Deary *et al.* 1989).

From this model of habituation, three predictions have been made:

1. More developed infants should habituate more efficiently than less developed. This can be either within an age group or across age.

2. Simpler (whatever that means!) stimuli should be habituated to more rapidly than more complex. Caron and Caron's (1969) study has often been quoted to support this claim. Here, an increase in complexity has been measured in terms of the increase in the number of elements in a pattern display.

3. If habituation is a measure of information processing, then it might be thought to predict other measures of information processing at a later age, e.g. intelligence, visuomotor skills, problem solving.

General support for this idea has come from a meta-analysis by McCall and Carriger (1993) across many laboratories. Of course other intervening factors have been suggested to underpin this association such as consistent maternal didactics. Bornstein (1998) has attempted to predict future cognitive ability from early measures of habituation, while partialling out the influence of the mother–infant dyad and maternal IQ, and found that habituation scores alone could predict later cognitive competence.

Nevertheless, no simple linear correlational model is likely to prove adequate in analysing the predictive value of early tests, and there is perhaps a danger in overinterpreting the early measures at the individual level, particularly in the case of children with clinical abnormalities. At best, perhaps, the measure can be used to look at changes in discriminative capacity with age, in an attempt to delineate the onset of newly functional attentional mechanisms with age in infants.

There is another serious caveat here. In interpreting individual differences in the rate of habituation it has generally been assumed that 'fast means efficient' but of course under some circumstances the encoding could be fast because *less* information had been taken in and learned rather than *more* information. For example, if there is extremely limited encoding—only minimal information processing is achieved (for example, the infant only encodes that a pattern is visible without encoding any details of the pattern) then we might get relatively rapid habituation, with short looking times. This might be accompanied by no post-habituation recovery because any pattern above visibility threshold will match the internal representation. This is the extreme case, but one can imagine that if encoding is the main limitation, then the assumption that rapid habituation signals more efficient information processing and higher intelligence, may be an extremely dubious one. For this reason, it seems only possible to use the information processing model in cases where discrimination between the novel and familiar stimulus is shown by post-habituation recovery. When this discrimination has not been demonstrated, rapid habituation may perhaps indicate fleeting visual attention (poor sustained attention), leading to poor encoding.

2.2.5 The Atkinson Battery of Child Development for Examining Functional Vision (ABCDEFV): a battery for assessing functional vision

Over the past 10 years we have attempted to produce a behavioural test battery, for measurements of functional vision, for both infants and young children with normal and abnormal development (Atkinson and Van Hof-van Duin 1993; Atkinson 1996). The battery was devised using ideas from paediatrics, ophthalmology, visual neuroscience, and developmental psychology, and included in the tests are a number of methods discussed above. To date this battery is normalized for mental age range from birth to 4 years, although an extension is being worked on for up to the mental age of 6 years. Of course, the chronological age of children completing the tests may be much wider than 4 years when clinical populations are involved.

Devising this battery was in part a response to requests from members of a number of professional groups [e.g. paediatricians, paediatric neurologists, developmental psychologists (clinical/educational), ophthalmologists, orthoptists, optometrists, teachers of the visually impaired] who might be interested in training in these methods and might find all or certain parts of the battery useful in carrying out assessments. For example, a reduced version of the test (without videorefraction or acuity cards) might be a useful starting point for any paediatric professional who is interested in vision but does not have the specialized equipment available. The rationale of these tests is that different parts of the battery tap different aspects of sensory, perceptual, motor, and cognitive vision, and combine questions about young children's vision which could be posed by parents, carers, teachers, and health professionals from paediatrics and ophthalmology. The battery is portable, so that it can be used in different settings. This battery is intended as a diagnostic starting point for pinpointing areas of concern in visual development in individual children and to help those involved in teaching and remediation. Failure on particular tests will not necessarily address the total extent of the problem, but rather raise a marker, so that the child can be referred to the appropriate place for more detailed testing and treatment when necessary.

The battery is divided into *core vision tests* (which should be possible with all mental ages and require no verbal responses or the motor ability to reach, grasp, or point) and *additional tests* (which are generally for mental ages over 6 months in conjunction with relatively intact manual skills). The tests are briefly described in Tables 2.1 and 2.2. Examples of the test material is shown in Fig. 2.5.

Failing many of these tests at specific ages may imply ophthalmological, neurological, attentional or general cognitive deficits (or some combination of these problems) and require referral and further testing in specific areas.

2.2.6 Photorefraction and videorefraction

The optical focus of a child's eyes will determine the spatial quality of the image on which most aspects of vision depend. It seems reasonable that the factors controlling development of the ability to change focus or accommodate and the process of emmetropization (the process whereby infants achieve a resting state of refraction which is neither long or short sighted and is like the average adult's refraction) must overlap and interact with factors controlling other aspects of visual development. What is more, refractive errors and anomalies of accommodative behaviour in infants are of clinical concern. In particular, they have been associated with the common problems of strabismus and amblyopia (see glossary for definitions).

The standard clinical method for assessing refraction without the need for subjective report (recognizing and naming letters) from the patient is 'retinoscopy' (sometimes called 'skiascopy'). This is a standard optometric specialist procedure, so will not be described here. Satisfactory retinoscopic refraction of infants and young children is possible, but requires high levels of skill, and extensive practice, specifically with paediatric populations. Most experienced retinoscopists consider 10–15 min as the maximum time available to carry out an examination on an infant or young child and will expect to get results accurate to about 0.5 D at best.

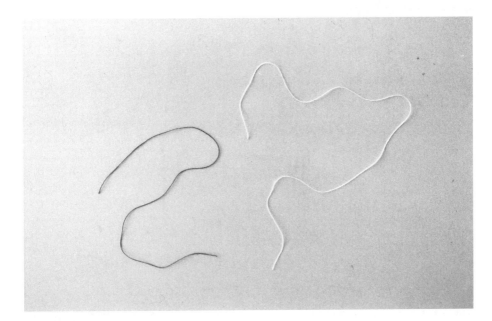

Fig. 2.5(a) (See next page for caption.)

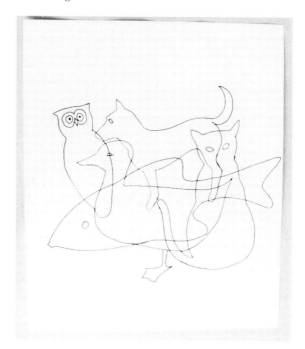

Fig. 2.5(b)

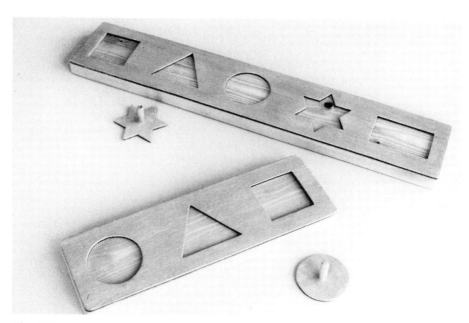

Fig. 2.5(c)

Fig. 2.5 Examples of the test material used in ABCDEFV. (a) Black/white cotton test. (b) Embedded figures test. (c) Two examples of the plain wood shape matching board.

Table 2.1 Core vision tests

Test	Purpose of the test
1. Pupil responses	To discover whether both pupils are responsive to light. Failure of pupil constriction in one/both eyes is likely to indicate severe neurological problems.
2. Diffuse light reaction	To measure a general responsiveness to light and dark (but not pattern vision). Only appropriate for very young infants and in cases of suspected total blindness. Failure is likely to indicate severe ophthalmological and/or neurological problems.
3. Symmetrical corneal reflexes	To measure alignment of the eyes. If eyes constantly mis-aligned (one eye turning in or out) misalignment is called manifest, convergent or divergent strabismus. May also indicate a marked refractive error in one eye, amblyopia (poor vision not due to pathology)/ocular/neural pathology.
4. Convergence of eyes to an approaching object	To measure whether the two eyes work together to adjust alignment for distance of fixated target. Failure to converge may relate to eye pathology and/or neurological problems.
5. Visual following of a toy to 3 m distance	To measure visual attention at moderate distance. Failure (for child older than 6 months) can indicate attentional problems and/or ophthalmological/neurological problems.
6. Peripheral refixation- lateral field testing	To measure visual attention and the extent of visual fields. Failure can indicate ophthalmological and/or visual neurological problems (such as hemianopia related to visual neglect). Age norms need to be applied to the estimated size of field to decide abnormality.
7. Defensive blink to object approaching face	To measure visual attention. Failure in child over 6 months indicates neurological/ ophthalmological problems.
8. Lateral tracking (saccadic or smooth pursuit eye movements)	To measure eye movements and visual attention. Inability to track (appropriately for age) may indicate attentional/neurological problems.
9. Visually follows a toy falling to the ground	To measure *object permanence*, i.e. the understanding that an object goes on existing when it disappears from view in children who cannot reach or grasp, but can move their eyes and/or head.
10. Acuity Cards (Teller/Keeler)	To measure visual acuity (described earlier in chapter 2).
11. Optokinetic nystagmus	To measure reflex eye movements. Abnormalities or absence may indicate subcortical and/or cortical dysfunction.
12. Isotropic photo/videorefraction	To measure accommodation/focusing, attentional shifts and refractive error.

Table 2.2 Additional tests

Test	Purpose of the test
1. Lang test of stereopsis	To measure stereoscopic vision (3D, binocular disparity, stereopsis).
2. Batting/reaching	To measure visuomotor development. Failure to reach in infants over 6 months indicates visual/neurological and/or visuocognitive problems.
3. Reaching and picking up black and white cotton thread	To assess fine hand and finger movement (development of a pincer grasp with opposition between the thumb and first finger). Also crude test of contrast sensitivity, when white cotton is used on a white table top.
4. Retrieval of partially covered object	Standard Piagetian measure of *object permanence* to gauge whether the child understands that an object partially hidden from view still exists and can be retrieved. Failure on this task in a child over 12 months may indicate visuocognitive problems.
5. Retrieval of totally covered object	Standard Piagetian measure of *object permanence* to gauge whether the child understands that an object fully hidden from view still exists and can be retrieved. Consistent failure on this task in a child over 15 months may indicate visuo-cognitive problems.
6. Retrieval with invisible displacement	Standard Piagetian measure of *object permanence*. It is more cognitively advanced than retrieval of a hidden toy in that it requires the child to understand that an object can be invisibly moved from location A to location B and still exist to be retrieved at B. Consistent failure in over 2 year olds may indicate visuocognitive problems.
7. Shape matching (special three shape or five shape board)	To test one aspect of spatiocognitive vision. Failure on task may represent a general delay or specific visual spatial problems. Test suitable for 2–4 year olds.
8. Embedded figures	To test one aspect of spatiocognitive vision. It involves segmentation of figure from ground together with shape recognition. Failure on this task may represent general delay or specific visuocognitive problems. Test suitable for 2–4 year olds.
9. Placing letter in envelope	To test one aspect of a combination of spatial, cognitive, and motor visual development. Involves relative orientation matching in space, combined with the appropriate orienting of the hand.
10. Copying block designs	To test one aspect of a combination of spatial, cognitive, and motor visual development. Test requires the child to copy various block constructions. The constructions have been graded in difficulty for ages 18 months to 4 years. In adults, failure on such tests is called 'constructional apraxia'.
11. Cambridge Crowding Cards	To measure acuity, crowding, amblyopia.

Because of the practical difficulties with infant retinoscopy, 20 years ago we began to develop various photo- and video photorefractor measures of refraction (Howland and Howland 1974: Howland *et al.* 1978, 1983; Braddick *et al.* 1979), finally developing the VPR1 (videorefractor) in collaboration with Clement Clarke International (see Figs 2.6a and 2.6b).

In many of the methods so far developed a small flash source is positioned close to the camera to illuminate the eyes from some distance away (e.g. at 1 m). If each eye is focused at the source distance then, in principle, the light will return from the point image on the retina, along its path, to the conjugate point at the source. If the eye is defocused, the returning rays form a diverging cone. The distribution of light returning from the pupils is recorded on film (photorefraction) or by a digital framestore (videorefraction). With either photo or video recording there are alternative optical arrangements for creating a light distribution which is dependent on the divergence of the returning cone and hence on the dioptric defocus of the eye. Many of the details of these methods and differences between them have been published elsewhere (see, for example, Howland *et al.* 1983; Braddick and Atkinson 1984). Later in Chapter 5, isotropic videorefraction is referred to in the context of emmetropization and methods of vision screening in infants and young children.

Photo- and videorefraction require much less co-operation from the infant or child than for retinoscopy. As attention is required only for the brief presentation of the flash, both eyes are imaged simultaneously. No lens or eyepiece is introduced close to the face, and head position is not closely constrained and these methods are well adapted to obtain refractive measures from both normal and clinical paediatric populations. The photo- and videorefraction instruments we have developed can be used throughout the age range from newborns (even premature infants) to adulthood. They can either be used in conjunction with midriases or cycloplegia to measure refractive error, or without either to measure the accuracy of accommodation or focusing at different distances.

We have included videorefractive measures in the ABCDEFV core vision tests, to measure accommodation, changes of focusing, and refractive errors in a wide age range of infants and children and in testing many clinical groups. Of course, individuals using this test need specialist training and equipment. The following would be a brief description of the procedure used with the VPR1 within the ABCDEFV battery:

'The child is seated on the parent's lap, with the child's eyes being 75 cm from the camera. The tester attracts the child's attention to a small noisy toy placed close to the camera plane, just above the camera. Usually a minimum of four flash video frames are taken in a dimly illuminated room to measure the focusing ability of the child. It is sometimes necessary to take a second series of four frames, with the camera at 100 cm from the child's eyes. The video images are measures off the video monitor and the focus calibrated by the computer attached to the video camera. Criterion values of defocus are taken as within the normal range for each particular age group.'

Poor changes of focus have been found in many children with marked clinical and paediatric disorders. Normal newborns can take up a wide range of focus, but on average tend to take up a myopic focus (within 20–70 cm distance), suggesting they

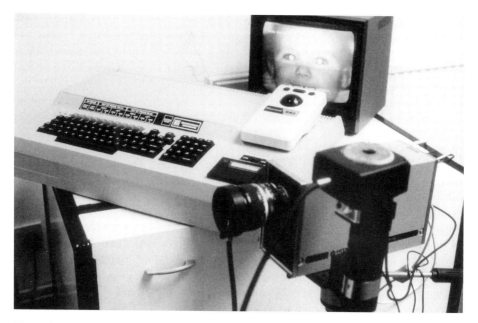

Fig. 2.6(a)

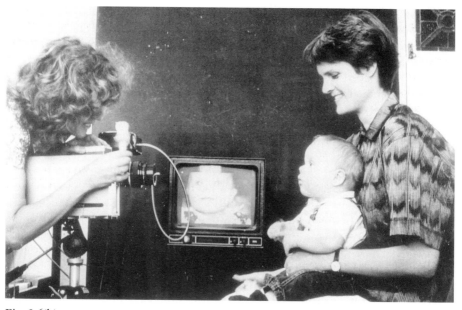

Fig. 2.6(b)

Fig. 2.6 Videorefraction: (a) apparatus for isotropic videorefraction, (b) infant being videorefracted.

are more visually aware in nearby space. By 6 months of age their focusing ability has markedly improved and they should be able to accommodate well on targets over the whole range of distances up to 1.5 m. If by 6–8 months of age the child is taking up a fixed myopic or hyperopic focus in either or both eyes, no matter what the distance of the target, then the observer should be concerned that there is a refractive error and/or an attentional problem.

2.3 VISUAL EVOKED POTENTIALS (VEPs) OR VISUAL EVENT RELATED POTENTIALS (VERPs)

VEPs or VERPs, recorded from the surface of the scalp and synchronized with visual stimulus transitions, indicate a neural response to a stimulus without a verbal or behavioural indicator of detection. They have therefore been attractive as a method of research on infant vision and for patients of all ages where motoric responses and verbal communication are either absent or limited. However, anyone contemplating this method should be aware (a) that the 'objectivity' of VEP recording is just as dependent as behavioural methods on the child's fixation behaviour; (b) that an active normal child of 6 months or more can rapidly remove scalp leads; (c) that the technique requires a high level of technical back-up.

The small amplitude and variability of the potentials recorded mean that the VEP signal can only be extracted by digital signal averaging. The general theory, techniques, and results of VEP measurements in adults and infants have been comprehensively reviewed by Regan (1989).

The procedures of electrophysiological recording can appear, to the infant's family, more unfamiliar and invasive than behavioural testing. A careful and sympathetic explanation of the procedure is especially important, especially to clarify the idea that electrical energy is being detected rather than applied to the child's head!

Electroencephalogram and VEP workers have developed systems, related to head landmarks, for specifying electrode locations, and with adult subjects frequently use montages of 16 electrodes or more to map responses across the scalp. Very little is known about how developmental changes in brain topography (or in the electrical properties of intracranial tissues) may affect these patterns, and the smaller size of the infant's head makes it harder to locate electrodes precisely. Montage-caps are a step that is being taken in some laboratories for ERP recording from infants (for review see Nelson 1994). In our unit we have usually used three electrodes for bipolar recording between an electrode over the occipital area, (about 1 cm above the infant's inion) and one on the forehead, with a third, reference or 'ground' electrode, either on the vertex or attached to the earlobe. The subject is only in electrical contact with a low-voltage preamplifier which is electrically isolated from the mains-powered amplifier. Details of these recording procedures are already published and will not be described here (e.g. Braddick *et al.* 1986*a*). If the child is anxious or inattentive the recording can be interrupted and the signal discarded on the current sweep. Separately averaged signals have usually been accumulated from interleaved presentations of different stimuli. A useful 'artefact rejection' filtering device has also been used to exclude sweeps containing any voltage excursion beyond a specified value.

If stimulus events occur at a rate of 1/s or lower, the measurable electrical response to one event is complete before the next event occurs. This 'transient' evoked potential has a complex waveform which changes markedly with age. This waveform has been assumed to be the sum of components arising from different stages of visual processing. If the stimulus events are repeated at 2/s or faster, the responses to successive events overlap, producing a periodic waveform at the frequency of the stimulus. This waveform is known as the steady-state VEP. The higher the repetition rate, or the younger the infant, the more of the signal power is in the fundamental and low harmonic frequencies; in some cases the waveform approximates a pure sine wave quite closely. In most of our studies steady-state procedures have been used, although in some studies of newborns transient VEPs have also been recorded. In much of our research using VEPs with infants we have been concerned simply with the presence or absence of a VEP response to a particular stimulus, or with the relative amplitudes produced by different stimuli. For these purposes, the steady-state VEP has advantages over the transient VEP. First, steady-state recording is usually more sensitive in practice. The power to detect weak signals depends on the number of repeated presentations ('sweeps') over which the signal is averaged. As each sweep is shorter at the high repetition rates used in steady-state recording, more averaging is possible within the limited time for which an infant remains in a good state. The value of this will depend, of course, on the frequency response of the response in question. While infants' high frequency responses are weak, they rarely get much larger for frequencies below 2 Hz, so the useful frequencies are mostly in the steady-state range. Further, the noise power generally falls off with frequency so the optimum is not necessarily where the signal is largest. Typically, signal averaging has been performed on between 25 and 300 sweeps; the square root improvement in signal/noise with number of sweeps, combined with the limited tolerance of infants for extended testing, brings diminishing returns for longer measurement periods.

The VEP response can only be identified in relation to a discrete, periodic stimulus event. Different types of event can be used to investigate different levels of the visual process; for example, an increase and/or decrease of field luminance ('flash VEP'), transitions between a pattern (e.g. grating or checkerboard) and a uniform field of equal space-average luminance ('pattern onset/offset'), and reversal of the contrast of a grating or checkerboard, i.e. substituting black for white and vice versa ('phase- or pattern-reversal').

In many of our studies we have wanted to examine VEPs elicited by changes in higher-order properties, such as stereo disparity, orientation, or direction of movement. However, it is usually impossible to achieve such changes without local changes in luminance and contrast, and so the VEP will include the response to these lower-order transitions. To isolate the effects of the higher-order property steady-state recordings were made in which the transition is embedded in a series of events that share its lower-order effects. For instance, changing the binocular correlation of a random-dot pattern necessarily requires changes to some or all of the dots, an event which would elicit a VEP even monocularly. The specifically binocular component can be isolated by changing the correlation four times per second (say) and by replacing the whole random pattern at a multiple of this frequency (say 24/s). The VEP component at 24 Hz must be assumed to arise from the dot changes, but components at 4 Hz and at the low harmonics such as 8, 12, and 16 Hz must be specific to the change in binocular relationships and so arise from neural processes combining the two eyes' signals (Braddick *et al.* 1980; Julesz *et al.* 1980). Analogous principles have been used to design stimulus sequences that isolate responses from orientation-specific (Braddick *et al.* 1986*a*; Braddick 1993) and direction-specific (Wattam-Bell 1991) mechanisms, and these studies are reported in Chapter 6.

Amplitude measurements have generally been used rather than latency. Amplitude measurements in transient VEPs depend on reliably identifying specified peaks and troughs in the waveform, and are very susceptible to noise at these extrema. Steady-state recording allows measurements that use more of the information in the signal. Specifically, the amplitude and phase of the component at the stimulus frequency ($F2$), and its harmonics can be extracted. For a small number of frequencies this can simply be done by multiplying the averaged waveform with sine and cosine terms; alternatively a fast Fourier transform can be performed. With increasing age, the higher harmonics of the VEP response generally become more prominent. Thus a measure based solely on a single frequency may be misleading, even in assembling data from different individuals at the same age. To alleviate this problem a measure such as $\sqrt{(F_2^2 + F_4^2)}$ is often used. The amplitude measured at any frequency does, of course, include an unknown noise contribution. However, a stimulus-related signal will have a constant phase, while the noise component at the same frequency will have a phase that varies randomly across 360°. The circular variance test has been used (Moore 1980; Wattam-Bell 1985) to provide a significance measure on the departure from random phase, weighted according to the amplitude of the signal in each sample.

2.4 CONCLUSIONS

Throughout this chapter many of the methods and techniques currently used have only briefly been described, with fuller descriptions being given elsewhere. In many of the following chapters particular use of these methods will be referred to without giving any details of the procedure. To answer many of the questions in visual development it is necessary to combine information across techniques and to develop even more sophisticated procedures for safe use with infants and young children.

3   Models of visual development

3.1 OVERALL THEORETICAL APPROACH

There are three major changes in visual behaviour in infancy, each linked to development in a different visuomotor or action system. The first most obvious sign of visual development in young babies is that whereas newborns do not seem to be very visually aware and do not use vision as a major sense for exploring the world, by 3 months of age infants are very visually alert. They look around seeming to choose what to look at and readily switch visual attention from one object to another. The second dramatic change in visual behaviour is seen in the visuomotor development of reaching, grasping, and manipulating objects. So far attention and exploration is in nearby space. Finally, with the onset of crawling and walking the third change is seen. The child extensively visually explores more distant locations and objects, crawls to them and then manipulates and investigates the objects in that part of space.

A comprehensive theory of visual development should be able to account for these three massive changes and their structural underpinnings within the neural system. Our neuroscientific models are not complete at present for either the adult visual system or its development, but are instead a set of partial theoretical accounts of some parts of the developmental process. Most of the ideas used in these models are from neuroscience, although important insights from the psychological 'representations' approach are sometimes incorporated.

3.2 NEUROSCIENTIFIC ACCOUNTS OF VISUAL DEVELOPMENT

3.2.1 Two visual systems in development: 'where' and 'what'

The starting point for our neurobiological theory of visual development is the idea of two visual systems, a phylogenetically older retinotectal system and a newer geniculostriate system. These two have been called subcortical and cortical, although the so-called 'cortical' involves the retina and lateral geniculate nucleus which are both in themselves subcortical. This model is schematized in Fig. 3.1. The anatomy of several distinct routes from the retina to the brain had already been identified in the last century and the visuomotor function involving the superior colliculus had been advocated by Cajal (1909), but the functional distinctions between the two systems were largely the result of pioneering studies in the 1950s and 60s, looking at the effects of brain stimulation and brain lesions (e.g. Sprague and Meikle 1965). Schneider (1969), proposed that the geniculocortical pathway was largely used for pattern discrimination while the retinotectal system mediated orienting responses in the environment; he distinguished between 'cortical blindness' in hamsters who lacked orientation discrimination and 'tectal blindness' in those who did not orient towards visually significant stimuli such as sunflower seeds. Thus the 'where' system was thought to control orienting responses and define 'where' an object is located to trigger foveation. Newer cortical mechanisms define 'what' is actually in the foveated area.

Using this idea, Bronson (1974) suggested a model for human visual development. In his model, newborn vision is totally subcortically controlled, with the cortex starting to mature at about 2 months postnatally. His evidence was based largely on the evidence on various newborn capacities such as visual orienting (using eyes and head movements) to track and foveate a large stimulus, coupled with the newborn's poor pattern discrimination. Advances in infant psychophysical methods and visual evoked potential (VEP) measures allowed Ol Braddick and myself to collect detailed data from infants. Hypothesizing from these data, our first theory of visual development was put forward in which distinct functional modules were defined, made up of linked subcortical and cortical brain networks. It was concluded that the neurological underpinnings of newborn behaviour were largely due to activity in subcortical networks, but over the first few months of life there was a gradual shift over to cortical executive control (Atkinson 1984). In this model, we used the idea from animal electrophysiology which is that certain areas have neurons which only change their response to certain changes in a particular visual attribute in the stimulus. So, for example, neurons in the lateral geniculate nucleus and superior colliculus are believed to give similar responses whether the visual grating pattern contains vertical

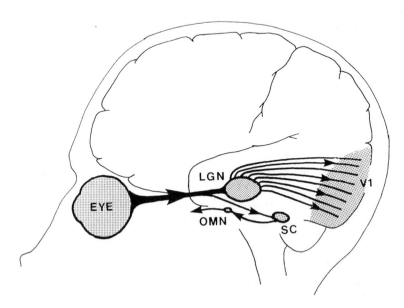

Fig. 3.1 Schematic of the two visual systems model. LGN: Lateral geniculate nucleus; OMN: ocular motor nuclei; SC: superior colliculus; V1: striate cortex.

or horizontal lines, whereas some neurons in the visual striate cortex will give a strong response to vertical bars and a poor one to horizontal bars and others will respond in the opposite fashion. We started to use 'designer' or 'marker' stimuli which were stimuli designed to isolate the specific responses of a population of cortical neurons, maximally sensitive to a particular visual attribute. For example, in orientation discrimination it was argued that if there was a clear change in behavioural response in an infant when the orientation of the lines was changed then that infant must have some basic brain mechanism working at a cortical level to discriminate between the two orientations. Of course, the conclusion from a lack of change in behaviour with a change in stimulus, should not necessarily be that the underlying discriminatory mechanisms are not functioning. A negative result always means that different ways of tackling the same question have to be devised and then the results compared across different techniques. This was exactly the way we proceeded in the 1970s and 1980s to arrive at the later theories.

Like Bronson, the key element of the Atkinson 1984 model was to hypothesize the emergence of cortical function postnatally, with the cortex taking over executive control from subcortical modules already operational at birth. However, cortical function was thought of as functioning of a number of cortical streams, each specifically processing particular types of visual information, each becoming operational at different postnatal ages, and each interacting with subcortical circuits to form distinct modules. This model forms the stating point of our discussion in Chapter 6 on cortical modules. In the 1984 model, there was still a broad divide into collicular functioning for orienting behaviour and cortical functioning for detailed pattern discrimination. There were still some unanswered questions about what was changing or developing so rapidly when occasional glimpses of behaviour was seen in the first weeks of life, which would seem to require a cascade of co-ordinated neuronal responses of the cortex, rather than the subcortex.

3.2.2 Three visual systems or streams of processing in development: 'where', 'what', and 'how'

Our theory of development in terms of two visual systems rapidly became at least three visual systems in the light of more recent infant data and in particular from ideas that were emerging in models of adult vision. The first of these models was based largely on primate studies in which cortical neurons, specific for particular visual attributes, were found to be clustered in anatomically distinct areas. Zeki and his co-workers were the first to define an area selective for motion information (V5 or MT) and a colour specific area, V4 (Zeki 1974, 1978, 1983a,b). This pioneering work formed the basis of the idea of multiple cortical modules in adult vision (Zeki 1993). Because much of this research concentrated on primates rather than rodents or cats, the new theories emphasized the role of the circuits within the cortex and reduced the role of the phylogenetically older subcortical tectal system. These theories postulated that both 'where' and 'what' responses were largely under cortical control, with the tectal loops being regarded as largely superseded substations for 'reflex' actions. Ungerleider and Mishkin (1982) put forward the theory of dorsal and ventral streams within the cortex, the two cortical streams being associated with different visual capacities. They suggested a largely parietal module involved in localizing objects within a spatial array and intimately linked to eye movement mechanisms of selective attention, and temporal lobe mechanisms tuned to the 'what' aspects of objects, such as form, colour, and face recognition. Supporting evidence for this split came from other studies on primates (e.g. Van Essen and Maunsell 1983; Boussaoud *et al*. 1990; Merigan and Maunsell 1993). Clinical observations of patients with specific focal lesions supported this dissociation between loss of position or movement perception and deficits of object recognition in particular patients (e.g. Damasio and Benton 1979; Zihl *et al*. 1983; Milner and Goodale 1995).

A second model, linked to the idea of a dorsal and ventral stream, was proposed for the adult visual system, based on the idea of two anatomically distinct streams, the parvocellular and magnocellular. The two streams are distinct morphologically at ganglion cell and lateral geniculate nucleus levels, project to different parts of primary visual cortex, V1, and continue within independent cortical streams to V4 and V5 (Van Essen and Maunsell 1983; Maunsell and Newsome 1987; Livingstone and Hubel 1988). The parvocellular-based system has been proposed to subserve detailed form vision and colour vision while the magnocellular system subserves movement perception and some aspects of stereoscopic vision. Van Essen and Maunsell (1983) suggested that the divide between 'where' and 'what' in the cortex could be largely as a result of the initial divide into parvocellular and magnocellular streams and popularized the easily remembered name, MT, for the medial temporal area (equivalent to V5) for the 'movement' specific stream as opposed to the 'form' and 'colour' stream via V2 and V4. Comparisons have been made between psychophysical data on adults and the functioning of the parvo-based and magno-based pathways (reviewed by Merigan and Maunsell 1993). We have made similar comparisons from looking at the time-course of development of specific cortical modules in infant development (which will be discussed in Chapter 6) There is some evidence to suggest that parvocellular-based systems may become operational slightly earlier than magnocellular-based systems (Atkinson 1992).

Many of the initial distinctions in sensitivity to different visual attributes, postulated for the M and P pathways in adults, have now been questioned by more detailed studies (for example see a review by Cowey 1994). It seems that some areas connect at a relatively early stage to both M and P systems. For example, V3, which contains many orientationally tuned neurons (for form information), projects mainly to the parietal cortex (for motion analysis). It may be that many of these extrastriate areas are not distinctive in their sensitivity to single visual attributes, but are much more specific for combinations of attributes, making up more complex stimuli. For example, cells in V4 may respond to colour rather than wavelength, and have mechanisms that allow them to mediate colour constancy (Zeki 1983*b*) and cells in MT respond to the global motion of a pattern rather than its component elements (Movshon *et al*. 1985). Nevertheless, it may be that complex deficits in vision arise in early developmental anomalies in these separate extrastriate pathways and that from these early deficits there are knock-on problems in analysing more complex stimuli. Chapter 9 will consider the deficit in relative motion processing, which has been found in many children with Williams syndrome. It may be a deficit in a relatively early stage of visual processing, yet may have effects on more complex visuomotor processing at later stages. A similar motion processing deficit has been hypothesized for dyslexics in VEPs related to the magnocellular stream (Livingstone *et al*. 1991), in elevated motion coherence thresholds (Cornellissen *et al*. 1995; Witton *et al*. 1998) and motion responses of area V5 as revealed by functional brain imaging (Eden *et al*. 1996).

3.3   MULTIPLE VISUAL MODULES WITH DIFFERENT FUNCTIONS

A somewhat different slant on the split between the function of different cortical modules has been put forward recently by Milner and Goodale (1995) who suggest that the distinction between the 'where' and 'what' cortical streams is not one for separating different properties, such as colour and movement, but rather two broad categories of visual coding with different functions. One stream is used for perceptual processing and one for controlling actions. As the ventral pathways contain specialized areas for face perception and the dorsal stream contains systems for controlling eye movements, reaching, and grasping, we can rename these systems the 'who?' and the 'how?' systems. One system helps us decide what and who we are looking at and one stream decides the appropriate responses and actions to be made on these objects. Rather than two distinct streams, Milner and Goodale[1] suggest multiple modules, loosely connected into two broad streams of processing, with each operating in an internal co-ordinated fashion. The relatively fast, dorsal, 'action' stream has a very short memory and is for automatic 'unconscious' immediate responses, whereas the ventral stream controls 'conscious' awareness and interactions with more long lasting elaborate memory stores.

Following on from the Milner and Goodale model, there is now substantial information about many of these distinct modules in primates. To try to summarize this vast literature would be a mammoth task. However, here an attempt has been made to schematize some of the important links found in primates which are likely to be important for different cortical modules in human adults and must be developed in infancy (Fig. 3.2). Further details of these modules are given in Chapter 8, Fig. 8.4.

Certain parts will no doubt need to be modified even by the time this book is published. Here I am indebted to the extensive reviews of Mel Goodale and David Milner and to Marc Jeannerod (1997). In reaching and grasping, Jeannerod has argued for a split in dorsal visual stream from the primary visual cortex to the primary motor cortex (MI). One route has connections between the parieto-occipital area (PO) and

---

[1] Of course this idea of *multiple cortical modules*, consisting of linked cortical and subcortical areas, is not a new one. For example in older studies, in kitten and monkey, visuomotor behaviour had already been dissociated into component visual channels with separate neural substrates for different action systems (e.g. Hein and Held 1967; Trevarthen 1968; Vital-Durand *et al*. 1974).

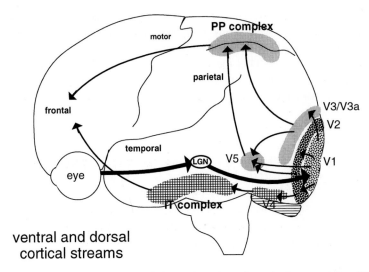

Fig. 3.2 Connections of cortical modules. LGN, lateral geniculate nucleus; IT, inferior temporal; PP, posterior parietal.

dorsal premotor cortex in area 6. Part of this route reaches the premotor areas directly and part relays within areas in the intraparietal sulcus (sometimes called the superior parietal module). This two-part system is important in the directional coding of movements towards objects. A second route from V1 to the motor cortex is via the dorsal extrastriate cortex to the ventral premotor cortex. These connections relay in the anterior intraparietal area. The system is responsible for transforming visual intrinsic attributes of objects into motor commands.

When these models are applied to human development it can be seen that it is not only possible to have differential timing of functional development between the two major cortical streams, but it is also possible to have differential development, internally, within different modules within each stream. In infants, the multiple 'action' modules within the dorsal stream controlling head, eyes, arms, hands, and general body movements each show their own developmental time-course. The first action module to become functional is the one used for making exploratory eye movements and for shifting attention through head and eye movements from one object to another seemingly 'at will'. The substrate for these head and eye movements are already operational at birth but change and improve dramatically in the first few months of life. This is followed in development by functioning in the action module controlling exploratory reaching and grasping. Next, the action module controlling independent walking starts to function. Of course early functioning in each of these action modules is not adult-like. It can take months or years for these systems to be identical to the adult brain modules. All these action programmes must involve some spatial analysis of the visual layout, but there may be quite different scales within spatial representations used for different systems. For example, for reaching and grasping the infant only needs a spatial representation of space which is relatively near to the body. However, this space may need to be extended if the child starts to use tools to extend the spatial area of control of the hands in order to manipulate objects at a distance. It is well known that relatively young infants, of a few months, can learn to operate a string that is attached to a mobile so that when the string is moved the mobile moves. This means that the infant's understanding of indirect causality is already present and the movements made near to the body (moving the string) is already associated with bringing about actions in more distant space. It is not possible to know from these studies to what extent we can stretch the distance between the hand and the mobile and still have correlated behaviour. For independent walking both peripheral vision and spatial layout some distance from the child must be represented to enable the child to find objects in spatial locations that are further away than arm's length. It is known that there are limitations to this understanding; however, from primate studies it seems likely that some initial perceptual analysis will be common to visual exploration, manual exploration and locomotive exploration. It could be imagined that the very early stages of visual analysis involve common pathways to V1 and early parts of the ventral stream, with the integration of this information from the ventral stream. The appropriate motor programmes and fuller spatial representations in the dorsal stream follow this early processing. It may be that for different action modules it is this integration which is delayed. Alternatively, we might consider that the spatial representations for modules which develop later are in some way more complex or involve integration over numerous subsystems for them to be effective. This is certainly true when we compare the reaching and grasping module with the one for independent walking. Vestibular and peripheral optic flow information must be integrated with elaborate co-ordinated leg movements, together with mechanisms for analysing depth and distance in a central field, for successful walking to a target. Whereas for reaching and grasping the peripheral optic flow information and vestibular information can be largely ignored while using depth and distance information in nearby space. For reaching and grasping, a spatial representation of the general nearby layout of objects will enable successful retrieval of objects, whereas both a detailed depth and distance map and a larger-scale spatial map of objects around the room will be necessary for a child to locomote to one part of space and retrieve the object, i.e. locate, travel to, reach, and grasp, in sequence. However, it is difficult to think of visual saccadic exploration and selection of visual targets using scaled representations of depth and distance, as being 'simple' in any sense. Once again the same depth and distance cues must be correctly interpreted to gauge the correct position and distance for the object to be focused on the retina and the eye movements to foveate an object, when shifting attention from one object to another, and must be precise if they are to yield useful information. Eye movement control systems are extremely complex and it is difficult to understand why, in terms of ecological validity, the infant in the first months of life has such an elaborate system functioning very similarly in terms of temporal parameters to the mature system in the adult, with relatively little visual input or learning being necessary to develop this system.

As well as these overt action systems, there must be internal covert systems of attention and memory. Here an imaginary line has been drawn between visual cortical modules for decoding incoming sensory and perceptual information and areas for categorizing and storing this information in visual memory buffers. This line is sometimes drawn between 'perception' and 'cognition'. However, the more we take on a neurobiological approach and consider the anatomical and functional connections and interactions between different modules, the more difficult it becomes to continue to make these distinctions. For this reason I have been led to abandon any serious attempt to divide developmental processes into 'sensory', 'perceptual', 'cognitive', and 'motor'. It is particularly in the area of *visual attention* that these boundaries are likely to be most imaginary.

3.4 DEVELOPMENT OF VISUAL ATTENTION

Traditionally, visual attention for adults has been viewed as a unitary, supramodal mechanism subserved by separate anatomical systems from those involved in sensory and perceptual processing (e.g. Posner 1980; La Berge and Brown 1989; Posner and Petersen 1990). More recently, two attentional systems have been postulated whereby a posterior one subserves spatial attention and an anterior one is involved in various complex cognitive tasks (Posner and Dehaene 1994).

A somewhat different model is that the same circuits are involved in both attention and sensory and motor processing. One approach to attention is to consider it a mechanism which enables 'selection for action' (e.g. Allport 1989), the action being either a saccade to fixate the object or a direct motor movement such as a reach, towards the object of interest. Such motor acts have been taken as indicators of a shift of *overt* attention, in contrast to *covert* attention when we attend to certain parts of the visual array without fixating or foveating the object of interest. Selective attention for spatial location would involve activity in a number of motor action modules such as oculomotor and those for reaching and grasping and walking (e.g. Rizzolatti 1983; Rizzolatti and Camarda 1987; Berthoz 1996). Selective attention for object recognition would involve areas responsible for object analysis (e.g. Desimone and Duncan 1995; Duncan 1996). Rizzolatti's premotor theory of attention is derived from neurophysiological studies of areas for coding space and from psychological studies of attention and orienting. Some parietal and frontal areas contain a representation which relates spatial representation, action control, and attention and ablation of these areas causes inattention (neglect) to particular parts of space. Inattention is accompanied by motor deficits, in particular motor movements related to that part of space. The cortical areas processing specific movements are controlled by other areas (e.g. the presupplementary motor area) and by certain subcortical areas (e.g. parts of the basal ganglia).

Reaction time studies of visual attention also support the premotor theory. When adults have to redirect their attention across the horizontal and vertical meridian they have to pay an extra cost in terms of reaction time with respect to reaction times for attentional shifts made within the same quadrant of space. This suggests that attention is related to motor programming (e.g. Downing and Pinker 1985; Rizzolatti *et al.* 1987). Another finding is that saccadic reaction times are dependent on where attention is located at the time of stimulus presentation (Sheliga *et al.* 1995). When attention was located in the same hemifield toward which the saccade was directed the reaction times were longer than when it was directed to the opposite hemifield. This can be understood as interference between execution of two motor programs: one is a motor program for the subject to covertly direct the eyes towards the stimulus and one motor program is for generating the saccadic eye movement itself. Support for the premotor theory has also been obtained in a later study by the same group (Sheliga *et al.* 1997) in which the effect of spatial attention on manual pointing and ocular motor saccadic refixations were measured, with the task being one of visually discriminating a peripheral stimulus. If attention was a superordinate system then we would imagine that it would affect both motor systems in the same way. In contrast if the premotor theory is correct then attentional effect would depend on the type of motor activity planned. As the task would cause foveation attention would be mediated in this case by the ocular motor system and should not effect the pointing task. Taken together there is strong support for the premotor theory from these results.

In the developmental context it is not possible at present to be in a position to decide between the two counter adult theories. However, it would seem that in some respects the premotor theory of attention is an easy one to go along with in development. We have evidence of attentional improvements in terms of reduced reaction times in ocular motor movements between birth and 3 months of age, when reaching and grasping systems are not at all well developed (Atkinson *et al.* 1987*a*). Information is also being gathered that suggests that there may be differential effects of attention on the preferential looking found in infants and their preferential reaching for the same objects (see Chapter 8). This is a preliminary result, but if substantiated would lend support to the premotor theory of attention. In terms of the present model, attentional systems will be considered as identical systems to those involved in motor preparation and execution which are already included in Fig. 3.2 for the adult.

This means that our theory of visual development involves a first stage with development of functioning in specific cortical channels, followed by development of integrative processes across channels within a single stream so that complete objects and people can have an internal representation. This is followed by the development of connections to allow actions to be made to this object or person. We can think of the first and second set of developing processes as taking part largely in the ventral stream, with dynamic on-line information contributed from the dorsal stream to add appropriate actions. Of course, integration between information regarding colour, shape and texture and information regarding movement must take place at a relatively early stage to enable separation of one object from another and each object to be separated from its background (figure-ground separation). These two processes of integration and segregation take place continuously and simultaneously, to provide smooth uninterrupted processing of a dynamically changing visual world. As yet there is not a complete neurobiological model of these processes in adult or infant vision, but recent results on 'structure from depth' and 'structure from motion' do start to address these issues (e.g. Kellman *et al.* 1987).

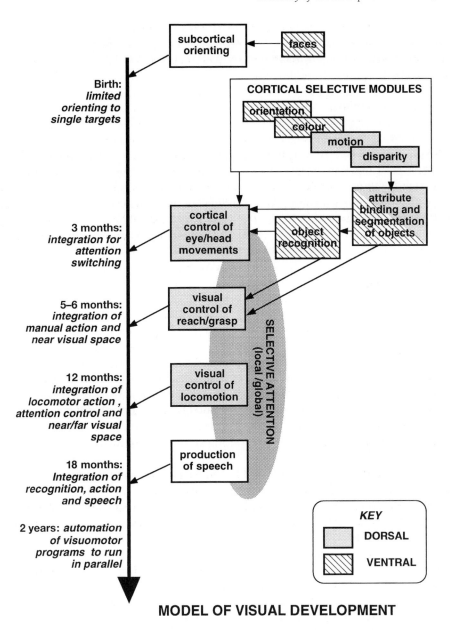

MODEL OF VISUAL DEVELOPMENT

Fig. 3.3 Schematic of current developmental model.

3.5 SUMMARY OF THE DEVELOPMENTAL MODEL

My model will be considered to consist of several overlapping processes discussed above, with some of the evidence being taken from developmental studies and the more speculative parts of our current knowledge of the adult system when it is damaged. The developmental model is schematized in Fig. 3.3. Each process together with approximate onset times in post-term age is given. In summary these processes are described below.

3.5.1 Crude orienting attentional system

This is the newborn's unconscious subcortical 'where' system for orienting head and eyes to abrupt changes in the visual world. The system is likely to operate supramodally and not be a specific system related to different modalities nor to different visuomotor systems. The superior colliculus is strongly implicated within this system, although there is likely to be a number of subcortical circuits involved in different responses. For example, newborn reflexive optokinetic eye movements made spontaneously to large field directional pattern movement are thought to be in part a result of subcortical circuitry involving the pretectum in addition to the saccadic eye movement circuits.

3.5.2 Functional onset of specific cortical modules

Here selectively tuned pools of cortical neurons become operational for processing distinct visual attributes such as relative size, shape, colour, pattern, depth, and movement. Some distinctions in timing can be made both in terms of onset of functioning and in relative improvements in sensitivity with increase in age for different modules. These timing differences may be taken to suggest models of differential plasticity at different ages for different subsystems. These timing differences may be taken to suggest possible differences in development of attributes related to largely dorsal stream functioning and to ventral stream functioning.

3.5.3 Development of integration ('binding') and segmentation processes

Here integration and segregation between and within subcortical and cortical modules starts to take place. This will involve integrative processes to combine information from different populations of cortical neurons to provide 'coherence' measures in motion, orientation, and disparity, to enable surfaces and shapes of objects to be defined. These processes allow infants to recognize objects as a whole and to understand the dynamic spatial layout of the visual world.

3.5.4 Integration of crude subcortical orienting systems with cortical attentional systems for control of directed eye and head movements

These processes are developed to switch attention from one object to another (parietofrontal). This will involve the disengage process to allow the infant to stop attending and processing one object and switch to another provided the two objects are in approximately the same depth plane. Interestingly, there are demonstrations that infants at about 3 months of age can show discriminative responses based on size and shape constancy mechanisms. For size constancy mechanisms to be operating the infant must be capable of using certain depth cues to judge the distance of the object and to scale up or down the retinal image size as well as identifying the object as the same object in two different points in space. These demonstrations would seem to suggest that relatively sophisticated mechanisms are already integrated within ventral object processing streams with dorsal stream mechanisms for eye movement control, by 3 months of age.

3.5.5 Development of reaching and grasping action modules

This process concerns the development of near-distance attentional systems for reaching and grasping. The infant develops initially crude arm extension and whole-hand grasp, and these motor systems must take visual information concerning the position of the object in space. This will involve discerning, at least, distance information, although initially this could be information from discriminating monocular depth cues rather than binocular. The uncanny coincidence of the initial discrimination of stereoscopic depth cues at about 4 months of age with the onset of more accurately directed reaching and grasping suggests that one system is readily linked to the other. Use of binocular disparity information implies that the object reached for has been fixated and this implies that there must be contiguous integration of visuomotor convergence eye movement systems with an action module controlling arm and hand movements. There is some suggestion that infants at this stage do not always foveate the object which they are reaching for, which might suggest that this integration is not always robust or even necessary for reaching crudely in nearby space. By 6–9 months of age normal infants are compulsive reachers for objects nearest to the reaching hand, although they may very soon afterwards show less reaching for an ungraspable object (such as a large surface). This suggests that, at the very least, crude object information about the relative size and distance of the object and the size of the infant's hand must be integrated soon after the initiation of motor programs for reaching, although again there may be brief periods where the object recognition and action systems are not synchronized. At one point in time the infant's object system may be more refined and developed than the reaching and grasping action system and this may be demonstrated by the fact that sophisticated discriminations have been demonstrated in preferential looking in infants at about 3–6 months of age whereas sophisticated preferential reaching is not demonstrated at the same age.

3.5.6 Development of locomotion accompanied by attentional shifting between different scales of representation of space at different distances

Although infants shift attention (as gauged through saccadic shifts) from one object to another in the first few months of life, they only shift attention from one object to another in *different* depth planes, i.e. from near to far distance, at a somewhat later age (beyond 6 months, if there is not a continuous visual stimulus linking the near point in space with the far). About the end of the first year of life, infants start to be able to follow an adult's point to reference an object of interest jointly, and this would seem to be good evidence of the infant's ability to shift scale from the adult's hand to the object in distance space. In addition, it seems that the infant is able to shift between different levels and scales of processing within a single object, e.g. local versus global processing in attending to a particular feature rather than the whole object.

There may be a stage in early crawling and locomotion when there is compulsive crawling rather similar to compulsive reaching. Whether there is true integration between recognition information from object recognition mechanisms for an object far away in distance space on the one hand, and locomotor programming for crawling on the other, remains an open question. There are studies which suggest that the infant's spatial representation of an object at a distance may be degraded or compromised by object processing of a prominent landmark in the same area of space as the object. Infants of 12–18 months have been shown to be unable to use a landmark to find a hidden object at a distance, whereas they can retrieve the object in nearby space (Bushnell *et al.* 1995; Hermer and Spelke 1994, 1996). Distortions of the attentional premotor programs to accommodate both the object and the landmark at a distance may be a partial explanation for this result. Retrieving an object from the opposite side of the room involves integration of processing information from at least four visual motor-attentional modules: (i) oculomotor systems for foveating, (ii) size and shape constancy object recognition mechanisms for knowing what the object is, (iii) locomotor programming to get to the object, and (iv) reaching, grasping and executing the actions when the destination is reached. The infant achieves all this by roughly 15 months of age, although the synchronous timing of these mechanisms may not be at all accurate until a later age. Parents often comment on inappropriate integration in 1 year olds who try to reach for passing cars out of a window and crawlers who overshoot the object of desire across the opposite side of the room. It remains a challenge for further research to look at these integration processes in detail in future research.

3.5.7 Integration of object recognition, actions, and speech

An action stream, that develops much later, is that for the production of speech, enabling the child to label objects and comment on actions of themselves and others. In early speech, and particularly in pre-speech, the infant often contiguously manipulates and explores objects or carries out rhythmic motor movements such as walking and jumping while making sounds. One of my best demonstrations of pre-speech is one of my own children Hugo, repetitively babbling in time to jumping up and down in his cot. This was pre-speech and not really communication (unless it was communication with the bedroom walls) as nobody else was present (I was hiding in a wardrobe with the tape recorder to record his speech, but could hear his jumping very clearly due to the rhythmic sound of the mattress springs).

Although I am not going to discuss the onset of the action module for speech, it is worth commenting on the very sophisticated visual processing which often accompanies speech. It is well known that newborns can make crude imitations of facial expressions, including imitating adult speech sounds. A more sophisticated form of imitation of facial expressions is seen at about 1 year of age, although the discrimination of facial expressions and speech sounds is demonstrated at a much earlier age. Given this early precocity, one of the strangest facts of human development is the late onset of speech relative to other action systems, such as reaching and walking. Discussion of language development is outside the scope of this book, but in a general neuroscientific theory of visual development the other major action stream for communication should not be completely forgotten as the two streams do not develop totally independently.

3.5.8 Automation of visuomotor programs and parallel processing

Throughout development visuomotor programs become more automatic as they become more adult-like. This enables the child to carry out two actions simultaneously and semi-independently, e.g. speaking and running, manipulating a toy and talking about it. In this model I suggest that this process is initiated at about 2 years, although there are examples at earlier stages of some types of parallel processing, where one action is semiautomatic and the other may be planned at the time of execution.

You will notice that throughout the brief discussion of this model there has been little mention of 'consciousness' and its development. Some psychologists would argue that the first signs of consciousness are seen in the infant's recognition that his or her own bodily actions are separate from the movement of objects around them. For Piaget, this would be the first stages of conscious self and existence of self and objects as separate entities. Others might argue that 'consciousness' is better demonstrated by 'metacognitive' tasks of 'theory of mind' at a later age (e.g. Wimmer and Perner 1983). As is becoming apparent in all the discussions of adult 'consciousness' in blind sight patients, the workings of many dorsal stream mechanisms seem to be largely 'unconscious'; only when we describe objects and recognize people do we show clear-cut 'conscious awareness'. Given that these discussions are largely unresolved in adult vision it would be premature to consider them in any detail developmentally.

3.6 CONCLUSIONS

In the following chapters only the first five processes of development of this model are considered, as this is where our unit has concentrated its research up to quite recently. We discuss the newborn's crude orienting system (process 1) in Chapter 4 and conclude that many subcortical visual systems, related to eye movement control, are already well developed. However, the infant seems to lack a reliably functional system for most of the subtle behavioural discriminations which we can relate to the cortex rather than subcortex. One exception may turn out to be in the domain of face perception, or it may be that crude configurational discriminations can be carried out by certain built-in specialized brain mechanisms, not involving the cortex. These areas have still to be found in subcortical systems and may involve the superior colliculus and pulvinar. Chapter 5 makes a slight diversion to optics and refraction, which are factors which may limit some of the pattern discriminations we measure in gauging acuity and contrast sensitivity and is an eye–brain system which undergoes continual development alongside development in the rest of the cortex. Chapter 6 returns to the model and process 2—onset of cortical function in specific cortical modules. This is a long chapter and contains a summary of a large part of our research in the 1970s, and 1980s. Process 3—integration and binding follows naturally on from this in Chapter 7, although this is not a complete account as yet of the multifaceted integration for object recognition carried out by infants. Attentional processes, linked to systems necessary for carrying out actions, which are process 4 and process 5 above are discussed in Chapter 8. Again this is a long chapter and contains a discussion of work on action systems for eye movements in shifts of attention and hand and arm movements for selecting objects to reach for and grasp. Much of this work was carried out in the late 1980s and 1990s.

Chapter 9 considers abnormality and plasticity for recovery in many of these five early processes. For the past 20 years we have always combined clinical research and assessment with basic research on normal infants. We cover a wide range of clinical conditions, with some relating to delays in early cortical functioning, while others are linked to attentional/action modules of cortex and subcortex.

4 Newborn vision

In terms of general development, the newborn infant's behaviour looks very similar to fetal behaviour in the late stages of gestation. There is one major difference: the newborn is moving and responding in air whereas the fetus is in amniotic fluid and consequently looks more controlled and co-ordinated. The slightly premature newborn, the term newborn and the 3-week postnatal newborn all appear similar behaviourally and somewhat limited in their visual responsiveness. It is difficult to get eye contact and they do not smile readily at visual stimuli. Hence many textbooks still state that the newborn is 'blind' and only slowly becomes visual after the first post-term month. Some neonatologists (for example, Heinz Prechtl) have indeed suggested that during human evolution it is possible that human infants born prematurely were more likely to survive compared with those born at term. The suggestion is that the evolutionary expansion of the fetal cranium was mismatched to the mother's pelvic size at one point in evolution. This would mean that large brained fetuses would have a harder time surviving birth as would the mother and that a genetic mutation reducing the length of gestation and triggering early birth had advantages for survival. There is at present missing evidence on prehistoric measures of infant head circumference and pelvic size, although a striking finding is that in no other existing primate species is their as tight a fit between pelvis and head size, nor are there the large numbers of premature infants, born to healthy females in the wild, in other non-human primates. What is obvious is that newborn human infants are extremely immature motorically compared with other non-human primates, and their postnatal development is comparatively slow. It has been suggested that the relative developmental rate is about 4 : 1 compared with the macaque; a month in the life of the former being equivalent to a week in the latter (e.g. Teller 1983).

4.1 STATE OF NEWBORN VISION: CRUDE ORIENTING

There is general agreement that the newborn does have some basic prewired representation of space. Crude localization movements to a visual or auditory stimulus has been consistently demonstrated when appropriate stimulus conditions are used. Newborns can be seen to slowly turn the head and eyes in the appropriate direction to the stimulus of a sound or light to their left or right in space. Others have claimed that newborns make more frequent pre-reaching arm movements for objects within their arm's length than objects at a greater distance than the length of their arm, and will bat at objects more with the left hand if the object is to the left and to the right if the object is to the right of their body in space. Of course, all these spatially appropriate actions are dependent on the newborn's motivational state and motor control, the former being labile and the latter extremely crude and inaccurate.

4.2 ACUITY AND CONTRAST SENSITIVITY

One of the most basic measures of visual development is that of visual acuity. One measure of acuity is called 'detection acuity' and this is the thinnest line or dot which can be distinguished from a uniform background. Now of course, if the line we are trying to detect has sharp edges we will still be able to detect something, even if it is seen with blurred vision. An edge can be blurred because of either optical blurring in the formation of the optical image within the eye itself or due to processes which degrade the retinal image within the neural system. Single dots or balls are often used in standard paediatric clinical tests of acuity, such as the STYCAR (Screening Tests for Young Children And Retardates) balls test, and give an approximate idea of what the child's real life limitations of detecting small objects will be under those particular viewing conditions (Sheridan 1969).

For measuring 'resolution acuity' the pattern used is often a bar or grating pattern. Again if we blur a sharp-edged grating pattern we will see fuzzy lines over some range of blur. If we optically blur a grating, where luminance is sinusoidally modulated, then as it is progressively blurred it will gradually fade completely into the background, finally disappearing completely from view and looking like a uniform homogeneously illuminated area. For this reason, sinusoidally modulated black and white grating patterns have often been used in comparison with uniform areas of grey, matched in mean luminance to the sinusoidal pattern, described in the preferential looking (PL) procedure in Chapter 2. The fineness of line for which the infant cannot distinguish between the pattern of stripes and the homogeneous field is taken as the estimate of resolution acuity. For sinusoidal gratings the retinal size of any single line is normally measured as the spatial frequency, i.e. the number of cycles (each cycle being one black and one white bar) contained in each degree of retinal angle subtended at the eye. Table 4.1 shows how approximate equivalences for spatial frequency measures can be given in minutes of arc, Snellen notation (both European metric and USA non-metric) and spatial frequency (in cycles/degree). A good rule of thumb is that your smallest fingernail's width subtends approximately $1°$ viewed with an outstretched arm at arm's length.

Many of the PL studies have yielded a rough rule of thumb for acuity changes with age—that is that the acuity (measured in cycles/degree) is equal to the post-term age of the child in months. This heuristic holds up to at least 12 months of age. Below there is a meta-analysis of the progression of acuity with age from average group data gathered from behavioural studies within our laboratory (see Fig. 4.1). This shows agreement with the above rule of thumb. From some studies there is a hint of three linear functions with different time constants covering the first period (from birth to 2 months), a second (from 6 to 9 months), and a third (from 9 months up to 4–6 years). There is some debate as to when adult values of possibly 50–60 cycles/degree for grating patterns are reached, but certainly single letter matching acuity values for 3 year olds can often be the equivalent of 6/9 Snellen letters (letter width of 1.5 min arc).

Data were compared using automated PL, the Teller cards, and Keeler cards for measurements of acuity in infants in the first year of life (see Fig. 4.2). In this study, the viewing distance across techniques has been standardized and all measurements

Table 4.1 Approximate equivalences between different measures of acuity

		Visual acuity	
Snellen (non-metric)	Snellen (metric)	Spatial frequency (cycles/degree)	Stripe width (min arc)
	6/3	60	
	6/4	45	
	6/5	38	
20/20	6/6	30	1
	6/9	21	
20/40	6/12	15	2
	6/18	10	
20/100	6/30	6	5
20/200	6/60	3	10
20/400	6/120	1.5	20
20/600	6/180	1.0	30
20/800	6/240	0.75	40
20/1200	6/360	0.50	60
20/1800	6/540	0.33	90

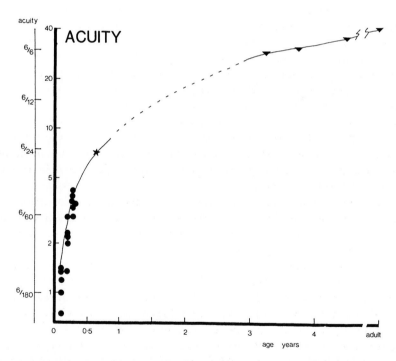

Fig. 4.1 Mean acuity measurements at different ages, from testing groups of infants in our Unit. The solid circles are data from preferential looking; the star is data from a tracking task test using a Gaussian-modulated grating; triangles are from grating orientation discrimination in an operant alley-running task.

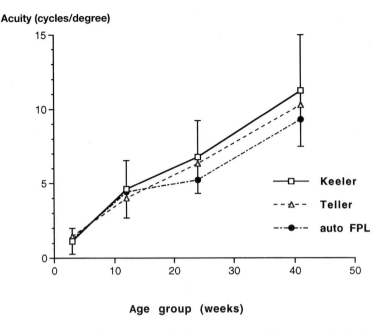

Fig. 4.2 Mean acuity data from groups of infants tested at different ages in the first year of life using automated preferential looking, the Teller cards and Keeler cards. The order of tests was counterbalanced across infants. One hundred and thirty-nine infants were tested. They were in four age groups: 0–6 weeks (mean age 4.29), 8–17 weeks (mean age 13.81), 18–29 weeks (mean age 22.37), and 32–52 weeks (mean age 39.82). In general the means obtained are somewhat higher than the published norms for Teller cards.

have been made by the same three observers using the forced-choice PL (FPL) procedure. From these results all three measures yield very similar results, with no significant differences being found between them.

A more extensive measure of the infant's spatial visual capacities is given by the contrast sensitivity function. The contrast sensitivity function is a plot of the infant's sensitivity to contrast (Michelson contrast) for grating patterns of different spatial frequencies, the resolution acuity being one value on this curve, i.e. the highest spatial frequency detected at maximum contrast.

4.3　MEASURES OF IMPROVEMENT OF ACUITY AND CONTRAST SENSITIVITY WITH AGE

Many estimates of contrast sensitivity, including measures of acuity, have been made in our own laboratory and in many other laboratories on both infants who are developing normally and in infants with abnormal vision. The detailed results of many of these studies have already been published and consequently only one or two studies from our own results will be dealt with here.

Our very first study in developmental vision (Atkinson *et al.* 1974) was to make the first published measure of contrast sensitivity on Fleur Braddick (our first child), when she was 2 months old. It was also a first for the new method, devised by Davida Teller, 'forced choice preferential looking', which is described in Chapter 2. Figure 4.3 is Fleur's contrast sensitivity function. Each point plotted is the result of many painstakingly careful observations made by Ol Braddick and myself on Fleur, when she was in a good mood, during the first few months of her life. The graph shows that the peak contrast sensitivity for a 2 month old is at best only 20% of an adult's sensitivity, and if the resolution acuity is extrapolated from this plot it is also very reduced compared with the adult. In this study the possibility that the reduction in Fleur's contrast sensitivity compared with the adult was due solely to optical factors (such as a marked refractive error) was dismissed because when Fleur was refracted only a very small astigmatic refractive error was found. We suggested that immature retinal processing and neural processing in the cortex must set the limits for the behavioural results. Since this first study there have been many measures of acuity and contrast sensitivity using the forced-choice preferential looking (FPL) method.

Many of us have also used the behavioural observation of optokinetic nystagmus (OKN) for stripe patterns of different stripe widths, and methods where either amplitude or latency of certain components of pattern visual evoked potentials (VEPs) have been measured. There are many reviews of different methods and measures (see, for example, Dobson and Teller 1978; Held 1979; Atkinson and Braddick 1981*a*; Norcia and Tyler 1985).

What conclusions can be made from all these studies? There is general agreement that there is a rapid improvement in both acuity and contrast sensitivity between birth and 6 months of age, followed by a steady increase up to adult levels by 5–6 years. However, estimates of acuity with different stimuli, different methodologies and different statistical measures may vary by as much as 2 octaves for any given age.

4.3.1 Comparison of acuity estimates from FPL and VEP measures

An age old debate has run concerning the comparison of VEP measures with behavioural preferential looking methods, with the persistent claim that the VEP method yields higher acuity estimates than do behavioural methods (see, for example, Banks and Bennett 1988). Even if it were ever meaningfully possible to compare statistically these two very different techniques, it is usually the case that the studies which have been compared differ in the infant populations and the size of group tested, the location in the visual field for the initial eccentricity of the stimulus and the size of the stimulus display. In studies comparing the two techniques, where adequate control for differences of subjects, procedures, and stimuli were made (Harris *et al.* 1976; Atkinson *et al.* 1979), rather similar estimates of acuity was found in infants (birth to 7 months of age). However, at least one well controlled study (Sokol *et al.* 1983) shows different values from the two methods and there are a number of others that also show discrepancies.

It is clear that certain stimulus factors can alter the acuity estimates. For example,

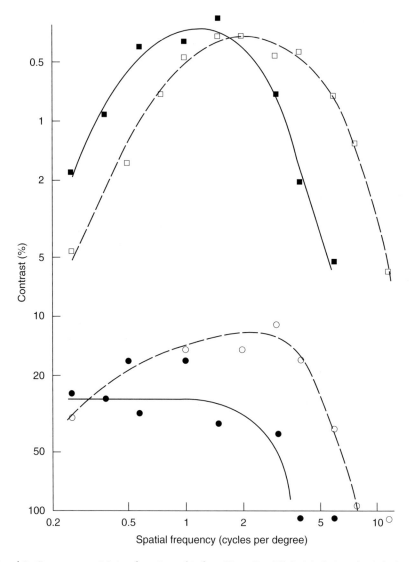

Fig. 4.3 Contrast sensitivity function of infant Fleur Braddick (circles) and adult (squares). Open symbols are for drifting gratings, filled symbols are for static gratings.

in Atkinson *et al.* (1983) it was found that acuity was higher if a screen size of 19° rather than 10° was used for a group of 1 and 2 month olds (all infants were tested on both sizes of the screen and the order of testing was counterbalanced with age and size of screen). The estimates of acuity rose by 2 or 3 octaves in the case of some individuals. Interestingly, there was no statistical difference in the estimates for the two screen sizes for 3 month olds. However, varying the eccentricity between 3° from centre field to the inner edge of the screen and 10° to the edge of the screen did not change the acuity estimates for the 1, 2, or 3 month olds. This is just an example of the interaction between factors which needs to be taken into account when comparing studies.

Nevertheless, there are some obvious differences between the two techniques which is likely to mean that there may not be identical limiting factors which need to be taken into account when comparing them. In PL the infant has to be in a state of calm alertness to enable the appropriate head and eye movements to be made repeatedly in order to achieve enough separate presentations for an estimate to be calculated (usually 15–40 presentations are necessary to make an estimate). In PL infants must be motorically mature enough to control the neck muscles to enable a head-turn and be able to make saccades reliably to the left and right. Infants must also have intact 'orienting' responses in visual space, i.e. to associate an interesting event in the left or right visual field with a behavioural response to the left or right. The reliability of the state of infants, their motoric control, and their 'effective visual fields' (i.e. the greatest eccentricity at which they will make a reliable orienting response to a visual stimulus no matter how large), all improve with age, alongside possible improvements in resolution. But how do we separate these different factors? Can we really do this?

It is clear that in many clinical conditions we cannot separate out these factors. Take an example of a child with very limited head, neck, and eye movement control who has severe cerebral palsy. It would be absurd to attempt to measure acuity accurately using normal FPL where we expect a reliable response in a few seconds. If such a child had reliable head orienting (but not eyes) then we might be able to use FPL and ignore the eye movements. But how are we going to know whether this non-speaking child can make slow but reliable head movements? We have often been in just this dilemma when testing clinical populations. Usually, you first try to find out whether they make reliable tracking eye movements for a conspicuous object, moved laterally from the midline. If they cannot do this then it is best to ignore eye movements during PL. Next you see whether they make reliable head movements to see a familiar adult who is standing in their peripheral field (the same eccentricity as the screens). If they can orient correctly to both the left and right, even if the response is slow and jerky, then you can often use these head movements to get an estimate of acuity. Usually you have to compromise over the number of trials, taking 10–15 trials as a maximum. Of course, for many children with cerebral palsy there are no reliable orienting head movements or eye movements and so PL cannot be used in its usual way. Sometimes these children have developed different response strategies such as hand tapping or eye gaze movements meaning 'yes' or 'no', so that they can be asked if they can see any stripes and these non-verbal responses used.

This discussion is not entirely irrelevant when considering normal newborns. Newborns vary constantly in their state, and state changes are paralleled by changes in alertness and muscle tone. This can make FPL a very variable measure in the first few weeks of life, as the infant is behaving like many of the older children with neurological deficits. Again this might be an argument for using VEP measures instead of behavioural in the very early months of life, particularly with children who have potential neurological deficits such as a hemiplegia.

However, in considering VEPs there are lots of other factors to be taken into account. When recording pattern VEPs the stimulus must be dynamic because only a dynamic stimulus will produce the necessary change in brain waves which is measured. In FPL the stimulus is usually static. This means to compare VEP and FPL measures both the spatial and temporal parameters need to be matched and we must

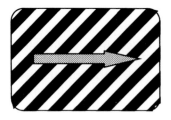

Forced choice OKN
Full screen grating drifts at 10.5 degrees/s, i.e temporal frequency = 1.5 Hz for oblique 0.2 cycles/degree grating. Direction of drift randomized left/right; 'blind' observer makes forced-choice judgement of the direction of infant's optokinetic nystagmus. Contrast varied according to observer's percent correct by a staircase rule, to determine contrast threshold (interpolated as the 70% correct level).

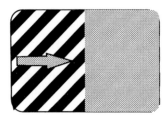

FPL (drift)
A drifting grating as for OKN fills half the screen, randomly left or right on each trial. The observer makes a forced-choice judgement of the infant's preferential looking behaviour, and contrast threshold is determined by a staircase similar to that used for OKN

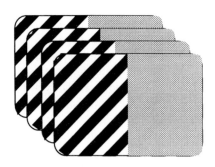

FPL (phase-reversal)
The same as FPL (drift), except that the grating is phase-reversed at 1.5 Hz (3 reversals/s) as in the VEP display.

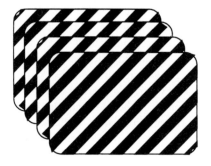

Phase-reversal VEP
The screen is filled with the grating phase-reversing at 3 reversals/s. VEP is recorded from midline electrodes (bipolar between occipital and forehead; indifferent on vertex; passband 0.2–100 Hz with 50 Hz notch filter). Signal averaged over 75–300 cycles for each of a range of contrasts. Signal amplitude plotted against log contrast is exrapolated to zero and the intercept taken as contrast threshold.

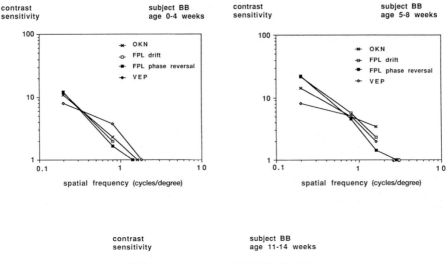

Fig. 4.4 A detailed comparison across different techniques for measuring acuity and contrast sensitivity in the first 3 months of life on a single infant, Ione, studied longitudinally. In this unique study (Atkinson and Braddick 1989) acuity and contrast sensitivity measures were compared using FPL, forced choice on the part of the observer for the direction of the OKN responses (FOKN) and pattern VEPs. Multiple estimates were made with the same infant and the same stimulus in the same location of the visual field. The stimulus was an obliquely oriented grating (at 45° with fundamental spatial frequency of either 0.2, 0.8, or 1.6 cycles/degree which could be either phase-reversed or drifted at 3 rev/s and 8 rev/s. Contrast was varied from 1.5 to 96%. The video screen subtended 58 × 47° at a viewing distance of 40 cm. The FPL drifting stimulus was spatiotemporally identical to that used for FOKN and the FPL phase-reversing stimulus used for the VEP measure. There were approximately 250 short interleaved testing sessions, balanced across conditions, in 15 weeks of testing. Extrapolated VEP amplitudes were used as the measure of threshold (as had been used in previous adult measures where a good correlation between VEP amplitude and psychophysical threshold had been found). The results at three ages are shown in the figure. It can be seen that the estimates increase with age in all four measures and that there is no overall difference in contrast sensitivity or acuity across the different methods. If anything the behavioural measures (FPL and OKN) gave slightly higher estimates than the VEP measure at the low spatial frequency (0.2 cycles/degree) and the VEP estimates were slightly higher overall in the newborn period for 0.8 and 1.6 cycles/degree gratings.

take into account the spatiotemporal contrast sensitivity function which also changes with age.

We have carried out one extensive study on our fourth child (Ione Biba Atkinson Braddick) in the first months of her life, to compare across techniques for the development of contrast sensitivity. The description, data and conclusions from this study are shown in Fig. 4.4.

4.4 FACTORS LIMITING ACUITY AND CONTRAST SENSITIVITY DURING DEVELOPMENT

There are at least four changes in underlying processing which are likely to be important when considering improvements in acuity and contrast sensitivity. These are changes in the optical properties and focusing of the eyes with age, differentiation of the fovea in terms of photoreceptor structure and density, myelination of the visual pathway, and increase in the number of synaptic connections throughout the visual system, particularly in cortical brain mechanisms.

It is of course possible that the primary limit on acuity and contrast sensitivity is in the optics of the eye itself. There are no marked optical aberrations in the cornea or lens of the newborn eye which would degrade the image and the optic media is clear at birth. However, focusing ability (accommodation) will also affect the extent of optical blur. From studies by Braddick et al. (1979) and Banks (1980) it is known that even newborns change their accommodation in the appropriate direction to focus on a nearby or distant target. This accommodation is sluggish and inaccurate but improves rapidly in the first few months of life. It is argued that because of the depth of focus (due to their relatively small pupils) of the newborn's eye, it is not possible for newborns to accommodate accurately. What is more, many infants have some astigmatism—a cylindrical component to the focusing of the image on the retina—so that lines along one axis are in focus, while lines along the orthogonal axis are out of focus. It was calculated that very large degrees of astigmatism (over 3D) could reduce acuity and contrast sensitivity even in the newborn, but as most infants show a relatively low level of astigmatism, this in itself is unlikely to be a major limitation. Further discussion of development of accommodation is in Chapter 5.

The morphology of the retina and the distribution of the receptors across the retina changes dramatically over the first few months of life (Youdelis and Hendrickson 1986). Several researchers have attempted to use the data available to calculate the imposed limitation which would be likely to result from the changing morphology (e.g. Banks and Bennett 1988). From these elegant models it seems reasonable to say that these peripheral changes provide one limitation, but would not alone produce the low contrast and acuity values measured in newborns and infants of a few months of age.

Myelination of the human optic nerve is proceeding for some time after birth, with rapid changes in the first few months until adult levels are almost reached at about 2 years of age (Friede and Hu 1967). There are data to suggest that pathways subserving subcortical vision are more advanced initially than cortical pathways and may be fully myelinated by 3 months postnatally (Yakovlev and Lecours 1967). From available data, the morphology of the dendrites of the lateral geniculate nucleus (LGN) are adult-like by about 9 months of age (Garey and De Courten 1983). During early development there is an increase in number of synapses up to about 8 months of age, followed by a pruning out period where the numbers start to decrease (Huttenlocher *et al.* 1982). However. this would appear to be a long slow decrease with adult numbers reached at about 10 years of age. Of course the processing power of the LGN and cortex depends not only on the number of synapses but the details of connectivity. This means that it is naive to argue that acuity depends on the maximum sensitivity of single cells found in visual areas, although it is likely to be related to it. Various researchers have shown that there is a general increase in single cell selectivity which is paralleled by increases in behaviourally measured acuity (e.g. work on LGN by Blakemore and Vital-Durand 1986).

The conclusion here is that it is not the optics of the eye which show a major improvement with age as much as the properties of the photoreceptors and the connectivity of central neural systems. The retina, LGN, and visual cortex develop in parallel anatomically. This means that maturation of cells in all these parts of the visual pathway are mutually dependent on each other, with the properties of cells lower in the system limiting those at the cortex. Improvements in acuity and contrast sensitivity, as measured by behavioural responses in monkey, have been compared with the highest spatial frequency response to which cells in the lateral geniculate and visual cortex respond with increasing age (Blakemore and Vital-Durand 1986). Acuity measured behaviourally is worse than the peak performance of neurons by a factor of approximately 2 at birth, but catches up gradually over the next few months. The upper limit appears to be similar in all levels of the system at about 1 year of age (Jacobs and Blakemore 1988). It is of course dangerous to accept the argument that there is a simple one to one relationship between the peak sensitivity of an individual neuron and the entire output response of the visual system. These comparisons merely serve to illustrate that there are interactive limitations at all stages of the system and that the input signal from the retina to the visual cortex is not adult-like at birth, nor is the synaptic processing within the cortex. In the case of human infants it is known from the very limited available evidence that the number of synapses increase between 2 and 6 months of age (Garey and De Courten 1983) It is inevitable that extensive interconnectivity with additional pruning is necessary to define the fine structure of receptive fields to achieve the adult values of acuity and contrast sensitivity. From the behavioural measures of improved acuity and contrast sensitivity in human infants and young children, this process would appear to be continuing until at least 3–4 years of age.

4.5 FACE PERCEPTION

It has been argued that much of the visual behaviour which is seen in the newborn can be accounted for by activity in subcortical visual systems. However, the single piece of evidence which perhaps runs counter to the idea of a non-functioning cortex is the finding that human newborns make differential responses to a face-like pattern (made up of three correctly oriented blobs for the two eyes and nose or mouth) compared with their response to 'non-facial' rearrangements of these blobs (Goren *et al.* 1975; Dziurawiec and Ellis 1986, de Schonen and Mathivet 1989; Morton and Johnson 1991). Goren and colleagues demonstrated differential head turning to the face whereas Johnson and Morton found that newborn infants tracked the face-like configuration further than the scrambled version of the same pattern. Using standard PL procedures, no marked preference for the face-like configuration has been found, but Ian Bushnell *et al.* (1989) found that newborns showed PL towards a familiar face in the first few days of life, representing very rapid learning of at least some facial features immediately after birth. Other groups have confirmed this result (e.g. Pascalis *et al.* 1995). The external hair outline feature seems to be critical to early face recognition. Some years ago, Ian Bushnell (1982) was the first to demonstrate the so-called 'externality effect' using photographs of real faces. In habituation experiments where two faces can be distinguished on the basis of multiple features such as hair outline, eyes and mouth, 6 week olds showed habituation recovery and thereby familiar face recognition on the basis of the external contour, the hair line. However if this cue was removed (Fig. 4.5) then the two faces were not discriminated until 3 months of age. This result has been confirmed by de Schonen and Mathivet in newborns (1989).

Extensive reviews of face recognition have been written by Maurer (1985) and Nelson and Ludeman (1989). Nelson has suggested that in the first few weeks of life recognition of faces is mediated by an early hippocampal-based memory which provides a 'snapshot' of the face. This system is unlike the adult system in that it does not allow comparison between one face and another, using a face 'prototype' for comparison. Only with functional development of the temporal lobe system after 8 weeks of age is the infant able to recognize faces in a similar way to the adult. A recent study (de Haan *et al.* 1998) suggests that infants have built up prototypes of faces by 3 months of age, but not at a younger age.

A debate remains on whether the newborn differential orienting response involves activity in temporal lobe areas identified in adults as responding specifically to facial stimuli. Evidence for such cortical specificity has come from neuropsychological patients suffering from prosopagnosia; this is the inability to recognize familiar faces with a remaining ability to recognize faces as distinct from other objects (e.g. Farah 1994); functional brain imaging studies revealing a 'fusiform face area' (e.g. Kanwisher *et al.* 1997); and electrophysiological recordings in non-human primates (Baylis *et al.* 1985; Desimone 1991).

Interestingly, Rodman *et al.* (1993) have presented evidence that the developmental onset of face-sensitive cells in the temporal cortex of infant macaques is at about 2 months. This seems to be rather later in development than would be expected on arguments from ecological validity, as it would seem important to have face recognition, particularly for familiar faces, developing rapidly around birth. In addition, recent studies suggest that a late component of the event related potential (ERP), known as P400, may show differential responses to upright versus inverted faces in 6-month-old infants (de Haan *et al.*, in press). The significance of this result is as yet unknown and

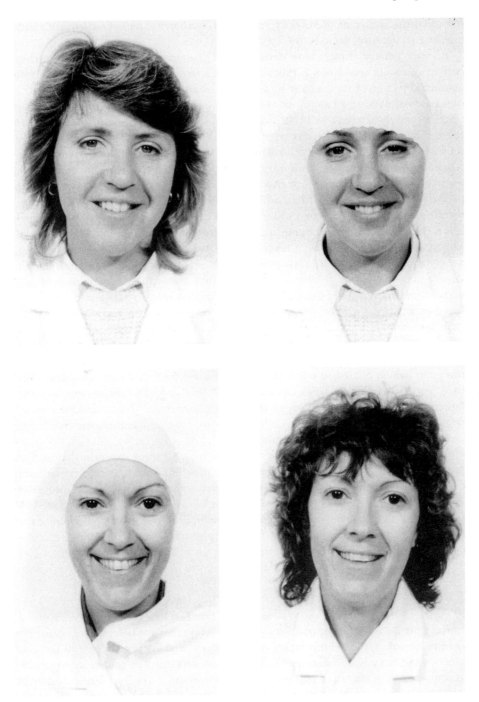

Fig. 4.5 Examples of the pairs of face photographs used in tests of the 'externality effect' in infants.

it could turn out to be a differential response to a familiar orientation rather than a genuine face recognition device.

Although many studies have demonstrated that newborns do not show a clear preference, using standard PL procedures, for a face-like pattern compared with a scrambled version of the same pattern, there is an additional piece of evidence which suggests that newborns have a bias for perceiving faces Using linear systems analysis whereby any pattern can be broken down into its component amplitude and phase spectra, Kleiner (1987) tested newborn infants for preferences between pairs of four different patterns. She took a schematic face pattern and a lattice or brick-wall pattern and using the Fourier transform of the patterns produced two composites—one with the amplitude spectrum of the face and phase spectrum of the lattice (which looks in the reconstruction to an adult like a brick wall in fog) and one with the reverse combination (which looks like a degraded face). She found that newborns preferred the composite with the amplitude spectrum of the face rather than the lattice. This result would support the idea that newborns are sensitive to the amplitude of the signal and insensitive to phase relationships in patterns (Braddick *et al.* 1986*b*) if it were not for a second result on newborns which showed that newborns showed a marked preference for the face-like stimulus with the correct phase and amplitude spectra compared with the 'brick wall in fog' stimulus which had the face amplitude spectrum but the lattice phase spectrum. This latter result implies that the newborn prefers the phase spectrum of the schematic face when the amplitude spectra are matched. There has been considerable debate about these results and the exact procedure which is used to normalize the amplitude spectra of different patterns so that they are matched in range (see Badcock, 1990, for further discussion). It seems difficult to interpret the results of the newborns viewing the composites, which appear to adults like low contrast, degraded versions of the objects represented by the phase rather than amplitude components.

In conclusion, it is unknown at present as to whether some subcortical area, such as the pulvinar, within some oculomotor orienting circuit may operate at birth and underlie the preferential orienting response in newborns. Tracking a stimulus further and for longer, which is the differential response of the newborn to the face-like configuration of three blobs, may represent an initial bias in the attentional salience system; this may in turn bias later face recognition systems to allow elaborate discrimination of faces and facial expressions in older infants.

4.6 CONCLUSIONS

In this chapter the starting point for visual development in the newborn infant has been discussed. The newborn makes fairly sophisticated eye movements in terms of kinetics and has a good orienting system, largely subcortically controlled, to enable examination of the foveated stimulus. This system seems to operate largely automatically and to be 'built-in' to the neural wiring circuits of the brain. The newborn system may be specially adapted to respond rapidly and to scrutinize certain ecologically valid stimuli, such as face-like configurations. However, any rapidly fluctuating, transient, discrete light source will alert the newborn and any high-contrast pattern (e.g. a black and white bull's eye) will hold their fixation well.

As will be seen in Chapter 5, visual development of many specialized cortical brain mechanisms is very rapid, particularly after the first 6 weeks of postnatal life. There is a hint of a period of newborn stability from some experimental data, as though the brain is recovering for a few weeks from the traumatic experience of birth, so that it can start to use incoming visual information at a more complex level in the following months.

5 Developmental optics—refraction and focusing or accommodation

In Chapter 2, the new methods of photo- and videorefraction for measuring accommodation and refractive errors in all ages of infants, children, and adults have already been discussed. Most recent studies on changes in accommodation with age have used one of this family of techniques. However, studies on changes in refraction (long- and short-sightedness) with age, where cycloplegia has been used to relax accommodation and look at the resting state of the eye, have generally involved retinoscopy—the traditional method of ophthalmologists and optometrists. In our current screening programmes, a number of different techniques, including photorefraction, videorefraction, and retinoscopy have generally been used and compared. Retinoscopy has been used as the 'gold standard' when considering refractive corrections in the form of spectacles, but we have used isotropic photorefraction and videorefraction for studying accommodative ability in infants and children of all ages.

5.1 CHANGES IN ACCOMMODATION WITH AGE

Newborn infants can show focusing changes in accommodation for targets at different distances in the first few days of life (Braddick *et al*. 1979; Banks 1980; Brookman 1983; Howland *et al*. 1987; Aslin *et al*. 1990; Hainline *et al*. 1992). However, to see this change in focus the targets need to be over 10° visual angle and to be conspicuous and relatively close to the infant (within approximately 1 m distance). The consistency and accuracy of accommodation rapidly improves over the first few months of life, so that by 6 months of age infants change their accommodation over a wide range of target distances (Braddick *et al*. 1979). The accuracy will depend on a number of factors: retinal and neural limitations on acuity, vergence responses, disparity detection, and chromatic aberrations; it is not certain what the critical limitation is at any particular stage. As young infants have slightly smaller pupils than adults they have a slightly larger depth of focus. Because of their reduced acuity compared with adults, they will often be unable to detect blur or poor accommodation in their responses. This means that their poorer accommodative responses prior to 6 months of age may be due to lack of feedback information concerning blur. In fact their accommodative range, over which their muscles allow them to change their focus, is enormous (30 D at least), so there are no physical muscular limitations in their system in early life. The eyes of a 1 month old infant will frequently be found to be focused at a distance about 50 cm, even when the visual stimulus is at a greater distance. Hence, the idea that young infants are 'myopically' focused. However, if accommodation is relaxed by cycloplegia, the average resting state of the infant eye is slightly hyperopic (1–2 D) with some astigmatism (a cylindrical component to the focus of the image on the retina so that if lines along one axis are in focus, lines perpendicular to this will be defocused by the degree of astigmatism).

Errors of focus found in older infants and young children accommodating on a target can be taken as strong indicators of refractive error and/or inattention (Braddick *et al.* 1988; Anker *et al.* 1995; Atkinson *et al.* 1996). In particular, many children with varying degrees of brain damage (e.g. children with focal lesions) show no change of focus for targets at different distances where cycloplegic refraction has already indicated that there is no marked refractive error. In these cases, it seems likely that networks involving accommodative mechanisms in conjunction with cortical systems have never developed normally in infancy. Whether this is due to damage to accommodative systems *per se* or whether it is due to more central damage to cortical attentional systems, cannot be determined from these measurements alone. However, in Chapter 8, measures of accommodation in conjunction with other measures of attention are discussed.

5.2 CHANGES OF REFRACTION WITH AGE

There are a number of reviews of studies on changing refraction with age in infants and young children (examples are by Baldwin 1990 and Howland 1993). Many are cross-sectional studies of clinical or selected populations, from which it is difficult to generalize about normal infants and total populations. Many studies of refraction in newborns report low amounts of hyperopia as the mean refractive error, with very little change over the first few years of life. This statement of mean refraction disguises the very marked changes in refraction seen in the early months for a small subset of the normal population and the marked reduction in astigmatism for many normal infants (e.g. Howland *et al.* 1978; Mohindra *et al.* 1978; Atkinson *et al.* 1979). To look at these changes in a relatively large group of infants has been one of the main aims of the two total population screening programmes we have carried out in the Cambridge Health District in the last 10 years with the help and collaboration of both public health teams and hospital ophthalmological groups. These studies are unique in making detailed screening measures on 70–80% of the total population in a birth cohort, but are limited in their generalizability across ethnicity because of relatively low numbers in groups other than Caucasian. These studies are very labour intensive and time consuming and not all of the data from either programme is, as yet, fully analysed. The screened populations in both programmes totalled about 6000 infants (7–9 months of age) out of which a large subset, including both infants who were normal and abnormal at screening, have been followed up to 4 years in the first programme and up to 6 years in the second programme. Fuller details of these studies are published elsewhere (Atkinson *et al.* 1984, 1996; Atkinson 1993, 1996).

The incidence of refractive errors and accommodative lag found in the two Cambridge screening programmes at 9 months of age is shown in Fig. 5.1.

Both programmes showed a similar incidence to a third population screened alongside the first Cambridge programme in Bristol in collaboration with my sister, Sue

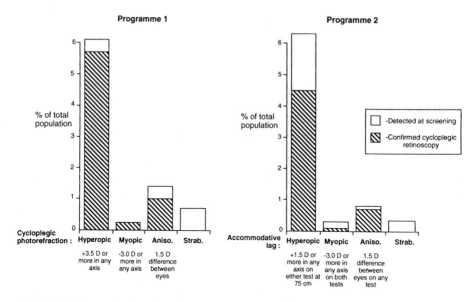

Fig. 5.1 Incidence of refractive errors (programme 1) and accommodation lag (programme 2) in the two population screening programmes in Cambridge. Aniso. = anisometropic; Strab. = manifest strabismus.

Atkinson (Atkinson and Braddick 1986; Atkinson *et al.* 1987). In the first screening programme, of 3166 infants screened in Cambridge at a mean age of 8.5 months, the mean cycloplegic refraction was 1.5 D of hyperopia, which included a degree of astigmatism for half of the infants. Very few infants (much less than 1%) were found to have large myopic refractive errors. A percentage of the population (4.6%) were found under cycloplegia to have significant hyperopic refractive errors (of 3.5 D or more in one or more axes), with many of these hyperopes showing marked degrees of astigmatism. Very few of these infants were strabismic at the time of screening (0.7% of the total population), with the incidence of strabismus by 5 years of age being between 1.5 and 2.5%. The accommodative responses of infants and children vary with the age and degree of hyperopic refractive error. Some infants may put in very little accommodative effort and suffer a permanently blurred input because of their hyperopic refractive errors. This is likely to lead to amblyopia. Others (with possibly lesser amounts of hyperopic refractive errors in early life) may have a high accommodative/convergence ratio because of their hyperopia, and this may lead to breakdown of convergence and esotropia. However, the detailed dynamics by which hyperopia leads to a disruption of this sensory-motor binocular loop is still only poorly understood. Other infants may develop an adaptive low AC/A ratio and accommodate without serious consequences and show good visual development or at worst, very mild amblyopia (which may include a meridional component).

Stress on the accommodative-convergence synergy from the necessity for large amounts of accommodation in hyperopic children, has been put forward to explain the clinical observation of the hyperopic refractions of children with early-onset strabismus. The implications of this relationship for ideas of visual plasticity are discussed in Chapter 9.

The possibility of countering any effects of early hyperopia on causing strabismus was tested in our infant screening programmes. In the first programme, in a randomized control trial of treatment with a spectacle correction for hyperopia, it was found that in infants whose hyperopia was corrected with spectacle wear, the chance of strabismus was significantly reduced compared with the uncorrected hyperopic infants who did not wear spectacles.

Further data and discussion of the different visual outcomes for different refractive groups, can be found in Chapter 9 when discussing plasticity. Here only the changes in refraction for the different infant groups who were followed up will be described. The changes of refraction that occur between 9 months and 20 months have so far been analysed in some detail (Ehrlich *et al.* 1997). There is a strong trend towards 'emmetropization'. The hyperopic refractive errors decrease; with the larger the initial hyperopia the greater the average decrease. Thus refractions tend to converge towards a common emmetropic value, although this average contains much variation. Of course many of the control children identified at screening are effectively very close to this emmetropic value at 9 months of age and so can only show small changes in refraction over this period in infancy.

As well as being hyperopic overall, many 9 month olds do have some astigmatism, which decreases with age (Atkinson *et al.* 1980). In considering the mechanism of emmetropization, we need to ask what is the proper way to express the data. A child with, say, +4 D in the vertical axis and +2 D horizontally can also be described as having a 'mean sphere' of +3 D and 2 D of astigmatism In the Ehrlich *et al.* paper the correlation between changes in these measures is considered. It seems that in the second description (sphere plus cylinder) the rate of change of these two quantities is independent of each other. In other words the reduction of the 2 D of astigmatism does not depend on whether this was combined with a large mean sphere or not. This is not what would be expected if mechanisms of emmetropization acted on vertical and horizontal axes separately. This analysis suggests that there is one process which controls the overall size and power of the eye to reduce spherical hyperopia—this might be driven by the detection of blurred images. An independent process seems to change the shape of the eyes towards being more spherical and less astigmatic. Our data from the first screening programme suggested that this second process acted more rapidly to correct astigmatism where the horizontal axis is more hyperopic than when the most hyperopic axis is in the vertical meridian.

There has been much discussion as to whether giving children a spectacle correction, and so reducing blur, may reduce the process of emmetropization. Our first screening programme has provided data which allows us to look at this question, by comparing the different refractive groups. Refractive changes in both the control group (infants who did not have a marked myopic or marked hyperopic refraction at 8 months) and those with refractive errors were compared for the first 3 years of life for changes in refraction with age (see Fig. 5.2).

There seems to be no significant change in the mean spherical equivalent of the

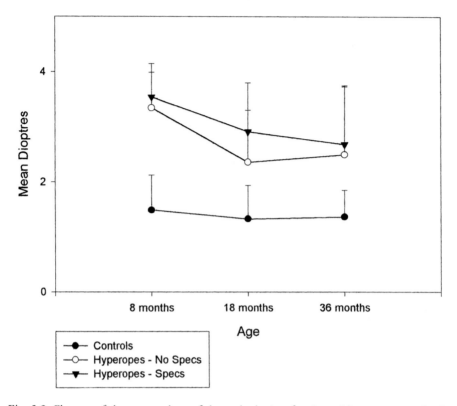

Fig. 5.2 Changes of the mean sphere of the cycloplegic refraction with age, measured using retinoscopy. Three groups are shown: (a) infants who at 8–9 months of age had normal refractions; (b) infants who at 8–9 months of age were hyperopic and were not given or did not wear a partial spectacle correction [infants with very high degrees of hyperopia (+6 D or more in any axis) are not included in this group]; (c) infants who at 8–9 months of age were hyperopic who wore, during infancy, the appropriate partial spectacle correction, to correct part of their potentially blurred vision.

control group's refraction between 8 months and 3 years, although there was a significant reduction in astigmatism with age in all groups. Most infants with small myopic refractive errors (see Ehrlich *et al.* 1995) and those with large hyperopic refractive errors emmetropized throughout infancy. Whereas those with small degrees of myopia appear to reach the same point in 3 years as the emmetropic controls, the infants with moderate hyperopic refractive errors in infancy are still significantly more hyperopic than the controls at 3 years of age. It is as though these hyperopes have not completely emmetropized by 3 years of age, whereas the majority of the population has emmetropized by this age. There appears to be no significant difference between those hyperopes with a partial spectacle correction and those who did not wear spectacles, in their rate of emmetropization. The latter is an interesting negative finding concerning the theory that changes in the rate of eye growth (and emmetropization) are dependent on the extent of optical blur present in the visual stimulus. On theoretical grounds it has been suggested that eye growth is likely to be largely determined by visual feedback, and that, consequently, the hyperopes who wear a correction should emmetropize at a slower rate (if at all) compared with the uncorrected hyperopes. Induced myopia and hyperopia, related to lens wear, has been found in a number of different species (e.g. Schaeffel 1993; Hung *et al.* 1995), although in general the results on primates seems more varied across individual animals and across the power of the lenses worn, than many of the results from other species, such as the chick.

It can be speculated as to why the spectacle wear does not appear to affect the rate of emmetropization in our infant hyperopes. Probably, the simplest explanation is that because a partial correction was used, and astigmatic errors were not corrected unless they were very large, the need for large amounts of accommodation to gain a sharp image was reduced; however, there is still a necessity to accommodate to some extent because of the remaining uncorrected blur in the partial correction. In our partially corrected infants, the accommodation required to obtain a sharp image is much the same as for the majority of children with normal refractions within the population. It has already been stated that from our outcome measures in terms of incidence of strabismus and amblyopia at 4 years, the partially corrected infant hyperopes (who wear their spectacles) show a significantly reduced incidence compared with infant hyperopes who are not corrected, so although emmetropization seems to have been relatively unaffected by treatment, visual outcome has been much improved by treatment. It is also interesting to speculate as to why the infants who were hyperopic in infancy are still more hyperopic at 3 years than the emmetropic controls. It is possible that nearly all hyperopic infants start in early infancy with poor accommodative responses (as is born out by the results from our second Cambridge screening programme) and that they remain variable in terms of their accuracy of accommodation throughout infancy. This variability leads to a poorer visual feedback signal than for controls, leading to a poorer signal for emmetropization. Whether this poor accommodation is a 'soft sign' for general delays in brain development in other domains (cognition and language) remains an open question. In a second, current screening programme, accommodative performance without cycloplegia forms the screening measure (see Anker *et al.* 1995). The outcome of children picked up in this programme, when available, may help us to identify the interactions of accommodation with refraction that create the risk of strabismus and the relationships between early visual development and motor, cognitive, and linguistic development in other domains.

5.3 CONCLUSIONS

There are many interesting questions as yet to be answered concerning the interaction of optical refractive factors with other aspects of visual development. It seems clear that most infants do not have a perfectly focused image of patterns and objects in the first few months of life, but as their neural systems of resolution are not mature either, this optical blur will be just one source of noise in the visual pipeline. Of course, failure of focusing mechanisms (either myopic or hyperopic) will become progressively more limiting as the child develops and uses information to decide their actions over a greater range of viewing distances.

Astigmatic errors in infancy (which are very common) will degrade lines in particular orientations and may provide distortions of shape. Distortion and blur might be expected to interfere with the operation of shape and size constancy mechanisms, whereby changes of size or shape in the retinal images of objects (due to viewing angle and distance) are cancelled enabling us to perceive objects of a constant size and shape. There are claims that shape and size constancy mechanisms can be demonstrated as functional in very young infants (even newborns). If this is true, then it is difficult to understand how these constancy mechanisms can operate effectively in the face of the distortion and blur in infants with high degrees of astigmatism.

As adults we are very aware of even minute degrees of optical blur and we are intolerant of it. However, we have argued that optical blur is unlikely to be the limiting factor in early resolution vision and indeed may not even be detectable by the infant in the first few months of life. Many other neural limitations of the system are present early in life and these are likely to contribute to the inaccuracies in early accommodation. In addition, many other visual attributes of objects, such as colour and movement, besides the clarity of the object's edge, its detail, and its overall contrast (which will all be affected by blur), are likely to be higher up the infant's attentional hierarchy and are therefore likely to be important in controlling the infant's responses to objects.

6 Functional onset of specific cortical modules

There is a rapid transformation of vision for infants between birth and 3 months of age. Often parents spontaneously comment on this. They see their rather sleepy newborn start to look around and eventually start to give real smiles and eye contact at about 6–8 weeks of age. This is followed by extensive visual exploration, attempts at verbal communication ('pre-speech'), and lots of batting movements with the arms at passing objects. Many groups have extensively studied infants over this transformation.

Our work has concentrated on indicators of cortical functioning, as it is believed that many of these changes in behaviour are related to underlying cortical functioning and executive take-over in decision making by specific cortical modules. This is represented in Fig. 3.3 (functional onset of cortical modules for orientation, colour, motion, and binocular disparity).

The main line of evidence for visual cortical development comes from considering the development of capabilities that require the specific kinds of stimulus selectivity that have already been found in cortical neurons in primate research. For example, certain cells give their maximum response to lines of a particular slant or orientation. Such oriently tuned neurons are found in primary visual cortex but not generally in subcortical parts of the visual pathways. A stimulus of oriented lines can then be designed to test out whether infants at a particular stage of development have such neurons operating. If it can be shown that the infants can discriminate between lines in differing orientations then it is reasonable to suggest that oriently tuned neurons are involved in the response and that those parts of the cortex containing many of these cells are operational. This has been called a 'designer' stimulus because the stimulus is especially structured to elicit a response from a specific population of cells. A second approach is to invent 'marker' tasks, where failure on this task is taken as a marker for a specific brain lesion in adult clinical patients or from animal lesion models.

By analogy, if the normally developing infant fails a task of similar design to the adult clinical task, then it can be inferred that the specific pathway found to be damaged in the adult, has not yet developed or is not yet functioning in the same way in the child as in the adult. For example, patients with a specific syndrome, called after Balint, have great difficulty disengaging attention from one object to shift their gaze and attend to another. Many patients showing this deficit have been found to have bilateral parietal lobe damage. If it can be shown that with a similar task infants have the same kind of difficulty as the Balint syndrome patient, then it is tempting to hypothesize that their problems might arise from circuits involving the parietal lobes. Of course this can only be a very tentative conjecture, and there are many other possible explanations. So failure of an infant on a so-called 'marker task' can start the investigation of a particular cortical module or process, but further more specific tasks will need to be designed to pin-point the exact failure point in the functioning of this circuit or module. Of course, ideally one would show 'double dissociation' in infant tasks, where the infant shows adult-like behaviour on one task (specifically designed for tuning in one cortical module) and failure on another task (specifically designed for tuning in a different cortical area). This type of result would suggest asynchronies in maturity of different cortical modules and not just a generalized immaturity in the infant compared with the adult, as may be the explanation when the child shows poorer results to adults on all tests. In the latter case, it is often tempting for the explanation to be given in terms of a generalized delay in development, or a motivational or attentional problem or even a failure of the child to understand the general task requirements in both tasks.

Using the rationale of 'designer stimuli' we have studied the development of systems for discrimination of orientation or slant, disparity detection, relative motion, and the disengagement processes of attention. The work of ourselves and others in these areas has been quite extensively reviewed (Braddick *et al.* 1989; Atkinson 1992; Birch 1993; Braddick 1993, 1996*a,b*), so only the main points which come out of these studies will be considered here. We have not carried out the development of colour discriminations in infants, although it is known that in adults a large part of the processing of colour involves the cortex. For writing the section on development of sensitivity to colour I am heavily indebted to the work of Davida Teller and her colleagues, who has been an inspiration to us all in this area.

6.1 COLOUR VISION

Fergus Campbell once said that he could never carry out an experiment on colour vision while William Rushton (renowned expert on colour) was alive and in the same laboratory—as Fergus put it 'he didn't have a licence for colour, only black and white'. William Rushton was known to be extremely scathing about young amateurs working on colour vision and so I guess I took note of Fergus's warning and this may be the reason why we have never attempted any studies on development of colour vision in infants.

In adults, visual signals are initially processed by the rods and three types of colour photoreceptors—the long (L), mid (M), and short (S) wavelength cones. These later inputs are combined into three postreceptor channels: the *luminance* channel that receives inputs from L and M cones; the *red/green* channel that receives opponent inputs from L and M cones; and the *tritan* channel which receives opponent inputs from S versus L and M cones. (For reviews see Boynton 1979, and Lennie 1984.) Of course, when a coloured object is perceived both the achromatic system and chromatic system are operating to give us the final percept and the brightness of an object cannot be consciously separated from its hue. This means that to say that if two patches of different hues are discriminated on the basis of colour, they must first be matched for luminance. This luminance match may well change across age. Many of the early studies have failed to eliminate the possibility of the infant making the colour discrimination on the basis of brightness (due to the stimuli not being equiluminant) rather than chromaticity. However, more recently, various strategies have been used to get round these problems, such as initially gauging the equiluminant point for each infant at each age, or varying luminance in conjunction with wavelength across a wide range, so that the equiluminant point must be included in the range. Anstis and Cavanagh (1983) devised an ingenious technique for measuring the point of equiluminance. A special computer-generated display was used to create apparent motion, the direction of which depends on whether stripes of one colour are more or less luminous than stripes in the other colour. The apparent motion elicits following eye movements, which can be observed in infants. When the two colours are equiluminant no motion is seen. Using this technique Daphne Maurer and her colleagues were able to show that the equiluminance point, measured in this way is very close for normal adults and 2–3 month olds (Maurer *et al.* 1989). Later studies have generally confirmed these results (Teller and Lindsey 1993; Brown *et al.* 1995; Teller and Palmer 1996).

Many studies of infant colour vision have been summarized in recent reviews (e.g. Teller and Bornstein 1987; Brown 1990; Teller 1997). Most of the studies have compared normal adult abilities with the infant's ability at different ages to discriminate between colours under different stimulus conditions. Nearly all studies have suggested that infants in the first month of life show poorer colour discriminations than older infants (e.g. Hamer *et al.* 1982; Packer *et al.* 1984; Varner *et al.* 1985). It seems that the test field size is an important variable, with the onset of the infant's responses to colour differences coming at a greater age the smaller the stimulus. There is still some debate concerning colour vision in the newborn period. Adams *et al.* (1990) found that newborn infants looked longer for a pattern of grey and coloured checks on a checkerboard than for uniform grey. This discrimination was not seen for a blue test stimulus. From this they concluded that newborns have colour vision for long but not short wavelengths. Brown (1990) has queried this argument because of the limited range of luminances used by Adams *et al.* (her claim is that a totally rod system could perform all the discriminations demonstrated in newborns by Adams *et al.*).

Banks and Bennett (1988) have argued that from studying the luminance and chromatic sensitivity of newborns, that from the ideal observer model the infant's detection of red–green differences is predictable from their luminance modulation thresholds. There is no differential loss of chromatic as compared with luminance sensitivity. However in the case of tritan stimuli they argue that there is differential loss of S-based cone sensitivity and this result can be used to argue for differential development of chromatic channels within neural systems within the cortex.

In early forced-choice preferential looking (FPL) studies, carried out in Davida Teller's group, 2 month olds were found to show a preference for all red stimuli embedded in a white surround, with the luminance of the red stimulus varied in small steps so that at least one of the red stimuli would be indistinguishable from the surround on the basis of luminance differences alone (Peeples and Teller

1975). This result can be taken as evidence of at least two functioning photoreceptor types, whose neural mechanisms can provide a discriminative behavioural response. Other later studies showed that 2 month olds could discriminate reds, oranges, greens, blues, and purples from white but failure to discriminate was found for certain greens, yellows and mid purples (Peeples and Teller 1975; Hamer *et al.* 1982; Clavadetscher *et al.* 1988; Allen *et al.* 1988). Further studies suggested that both red–green and tritan channels are functioning at 2 months and later. In a study of spectral sensitivity by Dobson (1976), infants were light adapted to reduce the contribution of rods. One to 3 month olds showed an elevation (compared with adults) in sensitivity for short wavelengths when measuring spectral luminous efficiency functions. Werner and Wootten (1979) studied dark-adapted infants and found that the spectral luminous efficiency curves for infants were similar in shape to the adult scotopic curve at wavelengths below 590 nm. However, all these measures could be compatible with a single functioning cone type. Pulos *et al.* (1980) measured the thresholds at 460 and 560 blue and yellow adapting backgrounds. Sensitivity was higher at 560 against the blue background and the opposite for the yellow background. This suggested that at least two cone types were operational; Pulos also found that 3 month olds showed an increased sensitivity to 460nm and postulated that infants are therefore trichromatic by this age.

Several investigators have looked at the time course of development of colour vision by studying longitudinally infants from a few weeks of age to several months of age. Morrone *et al.* (1990, 1993) found no significant visual evoked potential (VEP) response to an equiluminant stimulus consisting of a red–green reversing contrast pattern (with low temporal and spatial frequency) under 6–8 weeks of age (whereas Allen *et al.*'s, 1993, results have suggested a somewhat younger age for emergence of these responses). Morrone *et al.*'s results suggest that signals from different cone types do not generate a chromatically selective mechanism until about 2 months of age and in general the chromatic response for a low spatial frequency stimulus becomes mature before that to a high spatial frequency.

The temporal contrast sensitivity function for 3 month olds has been found to be band-pass in 3 month olds from FPL results for moving and counter-phase red–green grating stimuli (Dobkins *et al.* 1993), which is different to the low-pass tCSF (temporal contrast sensitivity function) found in adults. This has led to the suggestion that at 3 months the processing of temporally modulated red–green chromatic gratings might be undertaken by the magnocellular-based system rather than the parvocellular-based system for colour discrimination in adults. Further study of older infants and children is needed before these differences can be understood between early infant and adult functioning in colour vision discriminations. At the very least, these results suggest possibly rather different processing in young infants for dynamic chromatic stimuli than for large field static chromatic stimuli, a result which echoes our findings in orientation discrimination of static and dynamic grating patterns.

In conclusion, there seems general agreement from both behavioural and VEP measures that newborn and 1 month colour discriminations are weak or absent, given that adequate controls for luminance artefacts and chromatic aberration are used. Red–green discriminations emerge in the second month of life with tritan vision at an even later stage at least beyond 3 months of age. There seems to be general improvements in sensitivity at least for the first year of life (see for example Crognale *et al.* 1997), although there are few data on young children.

An intriguing and persisting finding from psychologists and paediatricians is that consistent colour naming, even of primary colours, is not found in children below 4 years of age. Nevertheless, colour names are often found in the first 200 words of a child's vocabulary at about 2 years. It seems that colour names are often used as a marker of attentional salience, with parents commenting that their child goes through periods when all 'interesting' objects are labelled with one particular colour name—usually 'red' or 'yellow'. We have no idea as to why young children show these idiosyncrasies. One challenge to future research is to understand why, although there is evidence for operational colour constancy mechanisms and fine tritan discriminations in 4-month-old infants, the linking of this highly developed discrimination system to the verbal communication system should be so many years later in development.

6.2 ORIENTATION

Following the pioneering cat and primate work of Hubel and Wiesel (1977), selectivity of cortical neurons to orientation differences has been found in many electrophysiological studies in a number of species. It is believed that orientation differences cannot be processed subcortically, except in circumstances where the signal is derived from feedback from selectivity within the cortex (e.g. Sillito *et al.* 1993).

In infant research there is now general agreement that normal infants, in the first few weeks of life, can discriminate between differently oriented static grating patterns, and as such this result can be used as evidence of some cortical functioning very close to birth. Our initial experiments on orientation discrimination led us to somewhat different conclusions, that discrimination of relative orientation developed postnatally starting about 6 weeks of age. In these studies a stimulus was devised that was a grating pattern which alternated quite rapidly (at 8 reversals/s) between two orientations, 45° and 135°, to which was recorded a 'steady-state' VEP response (this is shown in Fig. 6.1).

A significant 'steady-state' VEP can be identified as a repetitive signal at the same frequency as the transitions between the two stimulus patterns, with a consistent phase relationship to these transitions (Wattam-Bell 1985). A statistically reliable response at the frequency of the orientation change (or at harmonics of this frequency) is evidence for orientation-selective mechanisms. Such a response to an orientation change (OR-VEP) was found in 6–8 week olds but not in newborns (Braddick *et al.* 1986*a*).

However, using static grating patterns rather than dynamic rapidly alternating ones, both Slater and his colleagues (1988) and ourselves (Atkinson *et al.*1988*b*)

DYNAMIC ORIENTATION-REVERSAL STIMULUS

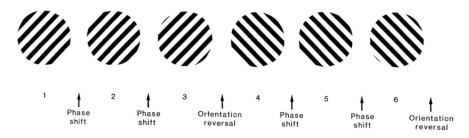

1		2		3		4		5		6	
	↑		↑		↑		↑		↑		↑
	Phase shift		Phase shift		Orientation reversal		Phase shift		Phase shift		Orientation reversal

Fig. 6.1(a)

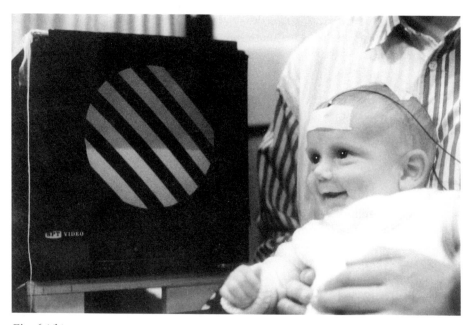

Fig. 6.1(b)

Fig. 6.1 (a) Schematic of the sequence for the orientation-reversal stimulus. (b) Infant ready to have his VEPs measured while viewing the orientation-reversal stimulus.

showed discrimination performance by newborns between gratings oriented at 45° and 135°, using an infant control habituation paradigm. In these studies the infant was first shown repeatedly a static grating pattern, of relatively low fundamental spatial frequency, oriented at 45° or 135°. When a pre-set habituation criterion was reached in looking times, the newborn was shown both orientations side by side. At this stage of the test it was found that on average newborns looked longer at the new orientation rather than the one to which they had been habituated, demonstrating relative orientation discrimination. Interestingly, newborns failed to show discrimination of these orientations if the post-habituation stimuli were *sequentially* presented, requiring the newborn to hold an orientation in memory after a single presentation and compare it with the next orientation presented (Atkinson *et al.* 1988*b*).

Following these results we have investigated how responses to orientation change vary with spatial frequency and temporal frequency, as these mechanisms appear to have different orientation tuning and temporal tuning curves at different ages. At a rapid reversal or switching rate between the two orientations (e.g. 8 reversals/s) and a fundamental spatial frequency of about 0.5–1.0 cycles/degree a significant response is found only in the second postnatal month and thereafter. With slower alternations (e.g. 3 reversals/s), the median age of onset for the response is 3 weeks postnatally (Atkinson *et al.* 1990; Braddick 1993). A typical result is seen in Fig. 6.2(a); the onset of sensitivity to orientation is shown in an infant tested longitudinally in Fig. 6.2(b). Interestingly, this rapid improvement in temporal sensitivity appears to be specific to the orientation response and not to non-orientational mechanisms. If the infant is shown a phase reversing (PR) grating, where the grating is in a constant orientation but the black and white stripes are periodically interchanged at 3 reversals/s or 8 reversals/s, a significant PR-VEP can be recorded for infants from birth. This supports the view that the OR-VEP is generated by a distinctive, rapidly developing, mechanism which is different from that responsible for the conventional PR response. Different ranges of temporal and spatial sensitivity have been found in

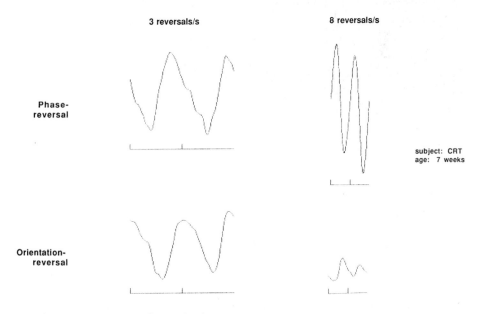

Fig. 6.2(a) (See next page for caption.)

Recordings taken from the same infant one week apart.

Age 2 weeks, 1 day...

A strong phase-reversal
signal occurs at 3 reversals/s:

but the orientation-reversal signal
at the same frequency is not
significant:

At age 3 weeks 1 day...

Phase-reversal responses are
still strong :

and now significant orientation-
reversal responses also occur :

Fig. 6.2(b)

Fig. 6.2 (a) Phase reversal and orientation reversal VEPs at 3 reversals/s and 8 reversals/s, showing spatiotemporal tuning. (b) Onset of relative orientation sensitivity in a 3 week old for reversals at 3/s.

the cell properties of the magnocellular and parvocellular pathways (Derrington and Lennie 1982). One plausible interpretation is that the magnocellular pathways are involved in fast temporal analysis, while the parvocellular pathways carry only slow temporal information. I have suggested (Atkinson 1992) that this may reflect that in infants the magnocellular-based pathways (needed for fast temporal analysis) may lag behind the parvocellular-based pathways (adequate for slow temporal analysis) in development. Further support for this idea comes from measuring the onset of infants' sensitivity to motion and disparity (see below).

Of course, infants' capability to discriminate between lines of different orientations is only one of the first stages in object analysis. It may be that the newborn has a system for registering a change of slant, but cannot combine successfully this information across orientation channels to segment an object from its background or another object. These secondary changes are considered later in Chapter 7. The sensitivity of infants to different degrees of orientation change was measured by recording VEPs while the infant views alternating gratings of different relative slants. It was found that generally the greater the difference in orientation, the larger the percentage of infants showing a significant VEP (see Fig. 6.3). This result suggests that orientation sensitivity is increasing rapidly with age over the first 3 months of life.

In addition we have used measurement of onset of a significant OR-VEP as an indicator of cortical integrity in clinical populations (e.g. very low birth weight premature

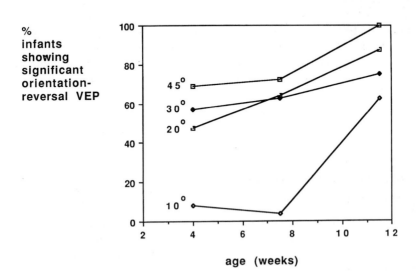

Fig. 6.3 Changes with age in the sensitivity to relative orientation as a function of angle between the two gratings.

infants and infants with perinatal asphyxia). Discussion of these results will come in Chapter 9.

6.3 DIRECTIONAL MOTION

Motion sensitivity is a ubiquitous property of all visual systems from the most primitive to the most advanced. In fact it has been suggested that in evolutionary terms, detection of relative motion is the primary method for breaking camouflage allowing segmentation of the visual scene. Given its universality, one might imagine that relative motion sensitivity is one of the first visual functions to become functional and indeed one of the earliest claims for young infants' vision was that they prefer to look at a moving rather than static display (e.g. Volkmann and Dobson 1976). However, this in itself cannot be taken as evidence of the operation of true motion mechanisms. Any moving stimulus also produces a temporal modulation and it is well known that infants show a preference for full field flicker, i.e. temporal modulation without coherent motion. In general, true motion detectors are in evidence if a differential response to different directions of motion can be demonstrated.

So what do we know about the motion detecting mechanisms of the newborn?

6.3.1 Optokinetic nystagmus—evidence for early directionality

It seems that the newborn does have a crude directional system already operating, evidenced by the optokinetic system—a stabilizing mechanism which is present in some form in the visual system of virtually every species. One of the smallest creatures known to show a visual optokinetic response is the zebra fish, about 1 mm in length. Visual analogues of certain clinical conditions, correlated with specific gene deletions, can be found in transgenic mutant zebra fish who show deficits in optokinetic nystagmus (OKN) (Chung and Dowling 1997). In humans, for binocular viewing, OKN can be seen at birth provided the stimulus is a full field, high contrast, low spatial frequency repetitive pattern.

The direction of motion matches that of the stimulus, which implies that directional motion mechanisms are present at birth. In newborn infants viewing with one eye alone, monocular optokinetic nystagmus (MOKN) can only be driven by a stimulus pattern moving nasal-ward (i.e. towards the nose), and MOKN is not elicited by movement in the opposite direction (Atkinson 1979; Atkinson and Braddick 1981*b*). Two mechanisms have been hypothesized from results of studies on the cat (Hoffman 1981); a subcortical system from retina to pretectal nuclei gives OKN for nasal-ward movement and a pathway via the cortex is required for OKN in the opposite direction (this is schematized in Fig. 6.4). In newborns, only the subcortical system is presumed to be operating, and is supplemented by the cortical system at about 3 months of age.

The results from a number of recent studies suggest that this subcortical–cortical changeover is not the whole story. These questions arise from studies on children who have undergone hemispherectomy, and from VEP studies using stimuli for direc-

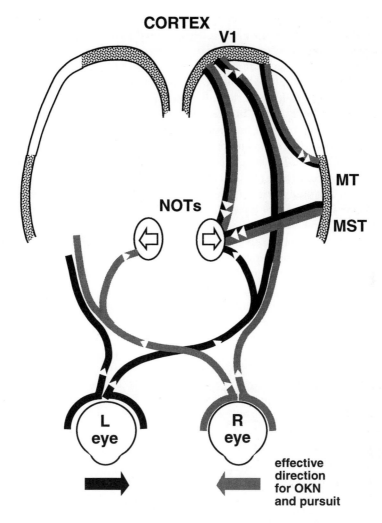

Fig. 6.4 Schematic of the pathways for OKN. Neural pathways to the nucleus of the optic tract (NOT); the brain is viewed from below. For clarity, pathways via the left hemisphere have been omitted, but are symmetrical to those shown. Pathways shown in grey carry information from the right eye; those in black carry information from the left eye. Each NOT is marked with an arrow showing the direction of motion to which it responds; this is the direction which in infancy or strabismus can induce OKN via the contralateral eye (as marked at the bottom).

tional motion responses. Both these kinds of evidence suggest that cortical mechanisms may be involved in OKN control at an earlier stage than that implied by the development of symmetrical responses, and that part of the early OKN asymmetry may be in mechanisms in the cortex as well as subcortex.

In our initial study on hemisphectomized children (Braddick *et al.* 1992) two infants were tested who had undergone hemispherectomy surgery in the first 9 months of life, to relieve intractable epilepsy caused by congenital unilateral mega-lencephaly. Both infants showed marked asymmetry of OKN with both binocular and monocular stimulation, with brisk responses to stimulus movement in the direction towards the decorticate half-field (i.e. good responses only for right to left stimulus movement for a child with the right hemisphere removed). This asymmetry is shown for one child in Fig. 6.5. In the direction towards the good half-field, the only response, if any, was occasional long tracking movements or reversed OKN. If a subcortical system alone was adequate to sustain OKN in children of this age, then with binocular stimulation OKN should be possible in both directions, as the subcortical systems of these children were intact on both sides. This result suggests that either the subcortical response is programmed to drop out once the cortical system is supposed to become operational (even in cases of a faulty cortex) or that there is suppression from the good cortex of subcortical responses on the other side.

Recently, we have had the opportunity to study a hemispherectomized child at an even earlier age, in collaboration with colleagues in Pisa (Morrone *et al.* 1999). By 10 months of age, this patient showed a similar dominance of OKN towards the damaged half-field, like our earlier patients. However, at 3 months, each eye showed OKN in the nasal-ward direction, like a normal newborn. This case supports the idea that a purely subcortical directional mechanism *can* operate in early infancy, independent of

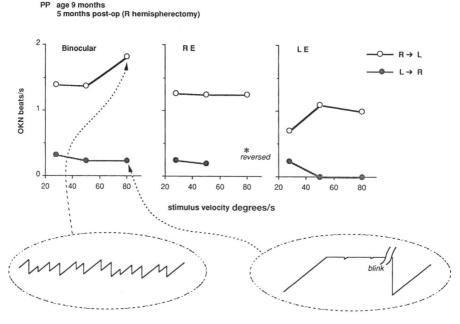

Fig. 6.5 OKN symmetry seen in a child who has undergone hemispherectomy, the right hemisphere being removed.

the immature or damaged cortex. However, this appears to be a transient stage of development: before the end of the first year OKN comes to depend on cortical directional mechanisms, and even if these are not working, the subcortical system can no longer sustain the optokinetic response.

Evidence on cortical mechanisms associated with the OKN response comes from asymmetries of the VEP to monocular movement. Norcia *et al.* (1990 1991; Norcia 1996) have recorded VEP responses to oscillatory displacements (90° phase shifts) of a vertical grating. In monocular viewing, young infants' VEPs show a prominent first harmonic response, that is a left/right directional asymmetry (a schematic of this is shown in Fig. 6.6a). The phase of this component is reversed between the two eyes implying that the asymmetry is between the temporal and nasal directions, as is the case in MOKN. We have recorded a similar response across a wide range of ages (Braddick *et al.* 1998*b*). These results, shown in Fig. 6.6(b), show quite large individual variations. However, there is on average a clear asymmetry at the youngest ages tested, which for the particular stimulus frequencies used has almost entirely disappeared by 5 months of age.

The VEP asymmetry persists to older ages for high rates of oscillation, which is again similar to a finding by Gesine Mohn showing that OKN asymmetry is present in older infants for high velocities but not for low (Mohn 1989). It is tempting to suggest that at least part of the MOKN asymmetry is not due to the absence of cortical processing but to asymmetrical cortical processing for moving stimuli. Once again these similarities may be deceptive. In a recent study in our unit, carried out by Alex Mason, where the amplitude of the VEP was measured separately for the two directions of motion we have found exactly the opposite asymmetry to the MOKN asymmetry (as shown in Fig. 6.7). In this case, larger VEPs are found in monocular viewing when the stimulus moves nasally to temporally rather than temporally to nasally (Mason *et al.* 1998). In addition, an important point to be made from our own observations is that the oscillating stimulus is not a good stimulus for eliciting OKN, nor can the result be due to an asymmetry of tracking eye movements (with more retinal slip in one direction than the other). Both asymmetries (in MOKN and monocular visual evoked potentials) remain a puzzle—they are contrary to each other and cannot at present be explained by a simple cortical take-over hypothesis in development. The suggestion might be that the cortical VEP asymmetry may be a mechanism to counteract the MOKN asymmetry early in life, and as the latter reduces so the cortical asymmetry reduces and eventually both drop out with complete cortical control taking over from subcortical control.

6.3.2 Directional discrimination and sensitivity

To test for sensitivity to direction of motion, a designer stimulus was devised that consists of a random dot pattern which oscillates vertically, its direction reversing four times a second. As direction reversals in an otherwise unchanging pattern could generate responses in mechanisms that are insensitive to motion, the pattern was modified so that a new uncorrelated pattern replaces the original pattern each time the direction reverses, producing incoherent jumps. These jumps will generate a

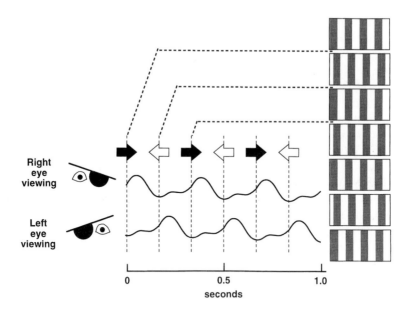

Fig. 6.6(a)

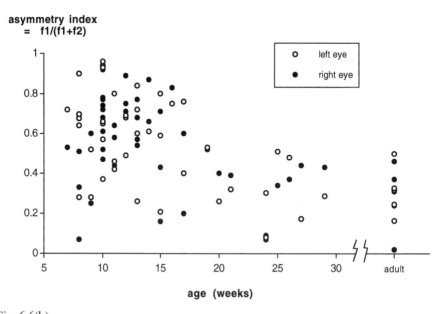

Fig. 6.6(b)

Fig. 6.6 (a) Schematic of the VEP motion asymmetry seen in young infants in monocular viewing. (b) VEP motion asymmetry in young infants. Each circle is taken from the VEP measure for an individual infant.

non-specific response and so, to separate in time the responses to jumps and those to true reversals of direction, extra jumps were added midway between reversals. This means that the 4 reversals/s are embedded in the eight jumps/s. We analysed the VEP to the jumps (at 8 Hz) and reversals of direction (at 4 Hz). John Wattam-Bell (1991), who devised this stimulus, found the first significant directional response at a median age of 10 weeks in normal infants.

Since this first study there have been many other experiments in the Unit, largely carried out by John Wattam-Bell, including behavioural measures of directional sensitivity by both FPL and habituation methods (reviewed by Braddick 1993 and Wattam-Bell 1996). The results are summarized in Fig. 6.8 The behavioural measures show a slightly earlier onset than the VEP measures at about 7–8 weeks compared with the 10 weeks found in the earlier VEP experiment. Before this age, the discriminative behaviour of infants shows no evidence of sensitivity to direction of motion, even though this may be reflected in OKN and related responses. Various questions can be raised about this finding, but they all seem to end with the conclusion that directional discrimination is absent before 7–8 weeks. The range of speeds for which infants can discriminate direction increases with age from 8 weeks, both in terms of the fastest and slowest speeds (Wattam-Bell 1992, 1996*a*). So very young infants might be sensitive within only a very narrowly defined speed range. However,

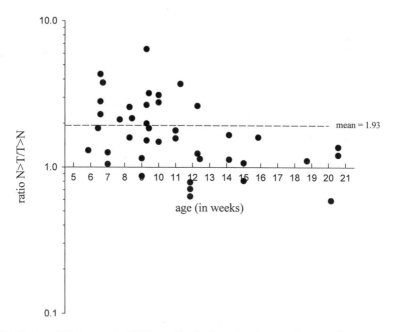

Fig. 6.7 Ratio of f1 harmonic VEP amplitude for stimulus moving nasally to temporally (N>T) versus temporally to nasally (T>N). The amplitude is significantly greater for nasal to temporal movement (*P* = 0.0001, paired *t*-test, two-tailed). Monocular recordings were made from 27 infants aged 5–21 weeks. The stimuli were sinusoidal vertical gratings moving unidirectionally at a rate of 3.125 displacements/s.

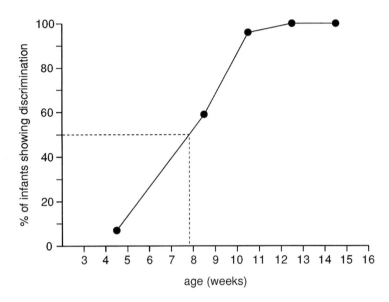

Development of direction discrimination (relative motion)

Fig. 6.8 Combined results of several studies showing onset of directional sensitivity in young infants.

systematic testing over a range of speeds has failed to find directional sensitivity in 3–5 week olds.

The behavioural testing by John Wattam-Bell (1992) depended on a preference for looking at a region of the screen where a figure appeared due to motion contrast at its edges. It is possible that this preference is absent before 8 weeks even though the underlying directional sensitivity could be present. However, infants showed a preference for a similarly segmented display, if the contrast was between static and moving areas, or between coherent motion and dynamic noise (Wattam-Bell 1996*b*). These discriminations require processing of dynamic stimuli and a preference for the segmented figure, but they can be made without directional sensitivity. John Wattam-Bell (1996*c*) also tested directional discrimination by habituation, as this method does not depend on an intrinsic preference. Again, he found that evidence for discrimination by 8 weeks, but not in 3–5-week-old infants, even though the younger group gave evidence for related but non-directional discriminations. FPL or habituation experiments with a motion-segmented targets depend on the visual system's ability to contrast opposed relative motions in two neighbouring regions. It is possible to imagine a developing system that could register the absolute direction in each region, but was unable to compare these in order to create a segmenting boundary. However, habituation experiments (Wattam-Bell 1996*d*) suggest that this is the opposite of the truth. The habituation experiments which showed discrimination at

8 weeks depended on detection of a motion boundary. Habituation experiments requiring sensitivity to direction *per se* (i.e. a region moving upwards in the habituation phase and downwards in the test phase) show discrimination only several weeks later. Apparently directional differences can serve to establish a perceived boundary before the direction itself becomes an interesting perceptual property for the baby. This finding reinforces the view that object segmentation is a primary function of the motion system.

6.3.3 First- and second-order motion

The discrimination of motion direction has often been thought of as sensitivity to motion energy (Adelson and Bergen 1985)—a concept from linear Fourier analysis in space and time which corresponds to the displacement of the bright/dark pattern across the visual field. However, it is possible to perceive motion when there is no directional motion energy. For instance, if a region of random flicker sweeps across an otherwise static black/white pattern, no peaks or troughs of luminance move in any consistent direction, but the sweeping disturbance will have a clearly visible direction. This perceived motion, without any motion energy that would be detected by a linear system, is called second-order motion (Chubb and Sperling 1988; Cavanagh and Mather 1989).

There is still much debate on what kind of mechanism is required to explain our ability to see second-order motion, but most investigators agree that it requires a distinct level or channel of processing from first-order motion energy (Wilson *et al.* 1992). Neurophysiological data make it likely, although certainly not proven, that second-order sensitivity requires non-linear mechanisms that operate in extra-striate areas such as V2 and V5, rather than in V1. Does this additional processing require further development, beyond basic directional sensitivity? We have investigated this in an FPL experiment, testing infants' preference for moving versus stationary flicker defined regions (Braddick *et al.* 1993, 1996*b*). In a first-order control condition, there were also regions of flickering and non-flickering dots, but the latter dot pattern moved coherently. A schematic diagram representing the stimuli used is shown in Fig. 6.9.

Infants aged 8–10 weeks, as well as those aged 16–20 weeks, showed a preference for the moving area in both first- and second-order displays. This preference increased with age, and was stronger with first-order motion at both ages, but showed no sign of differential development of first- and second-order sensitivity. Although there is a good deal of adult psychophysical evidence that separate pathways are required for the two forms of motion (see, for example, Ledgway and Smith 1994; Mather and West 1993), developmentally they seem to follow the same course. One possible explanation of this would be if the limit on the behavioural measures of infant motion sensitivity was set by a common path for the two motion signals, rather than at an earlier stage where they are processed separately. That is, experiments on infants' behavioural motion sensitivity may reveal development of extra-striate motion pathways, rather than the primary cortical directionality which feeds them. If so, this would make it easier to understand any discrepancy between OKN

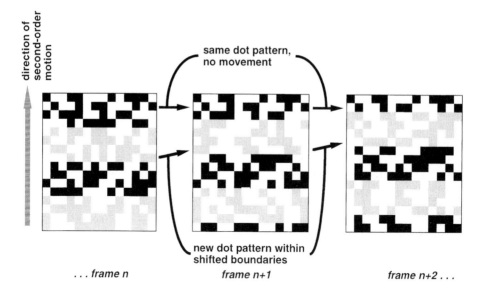

direction of second-order motion

same dot pattern, no movement

new dot pattern within shifted boundaries

... frame n   frame n+1   frame n+2 ...

second-order motion display

Fig. 6.9 Schematic diagram of the second-order stimulus used in our infant experiments.

and motion-asymmetry evidence on the one hand, and directional discrimination on the other—the two kinds of processing may use divergent pathways from V1. But, as can be seen from functional magnetic resonance imaging data, the cortical motion pathway is a complex one, and there is a long way to go before the development of its multiple functional areas can be fully understood.

6.3.4 Conclusions on motion

One of the main uses of relative motion information is to segment an object from its background and to separate one object from another. For this reason this whole section on development of mechanisms for detecting relative motion could have been placed in the chapter under object perception. However, it seems more appropriate to consider it here as a primary cortical system underpinning all other more complex pieces of visual processing. However, the motion processing story can be taken further; while considering in Chapter 7 (object perception) the development of sensitivity to motion coherence, where local, and global, processing must take place over extended regions of the visual field. The observer must learn to ignore random movements of elements within one region and amalgamate other elements, with common movement, into a bounded region. These coherence thresholds will be returned to when the unusual development of children with Williams syndrome is considered in Chapter 9.

6.4 BINOCULARITY

Any response dependent on detection of binocular correlation or disparity must be dependent on the operation of cortical rather than subcortical mechanisms, as the signals from the two eyes interact for the first time in striate cortex. It is known from extensive neurophysiological studies on cats and primates that the input signal from the lateral geniculate nucleus to the visual cortex is separate for the two eyes, with cells in layer IV of the cortex being organized into ocular dominance columns. The ocular dominance columns form stripes within V1, with one set of cells in one column being monocularly driven by one eye and cells in the column next to it being monocularly driven by the other eye. Outside layer IV cells in other cortical layers are largely binocularly driven. Ocular dominance columns have been found in primates at or shortly after birth, but the binocular connections are generally thought to become tuned postnatally in all primates, including humans. The plasticity of these binocular connections within the cortex has formed the basis of all the early measures of critical periods, and this plasticity will be discussed further in Chapter 9.

There are now a great many studies on onset of binocular responses in human infants. In our first study in Lew Lipsitt's lab we demonstrated such a response using a sucking habituation paradigm (Atkinson and Braddick 1976), finding that some 2–3 month olds showed sucking dishabituation to a random dot stereogram containing a square, identifiable by disparity detection. In a second major group of studies on binocularity in infants we used the ingenious technology of Bela Julesz. VEPs were recorded in infants who watched a dynamic random-dot correlogram (Braddick *et al.* 1980; Julesz *et al.* 1980). This display consists of a random pattern of red and green dots which are changed completely on each video frame. Two phases alternate: in one the red and green dot patterns are identical (correlated), and in the other the green pattern is the negative of the red (anticorrelated). The infant wears custom-made red–green goggles (see Fig. 6.10a).

Each eye individually sees a pattern in which the alternations are undetectable, as the pattern change at alternation is no different from that which occurs on every other frame. However, cortical neurons which integrate signals from the two eyes will respond to the difference between the correlated display that can be fused perfectly, and the uncorrelated display which cannot. This response can be detected as a periodic VEP at the alternation frequency, whose emergence can be tracked longitudinally in individual infants (Braddick *et al.* 1983; Wattam-Bell *et al.* 1987). It was found that the correlogram VEP response was seen first at some age between 8 and 20 weeks, normally between 11 and 16 weeks, in individual infants (shown in Fig. 6.10b).

The findings are not closely dependent on how the infant's response to correlation–anticorrelation is measured. Similar displays can be used in a FPL test: one-half of the display remains uniformly anticorrelated, while the other half contains large checks which alternate between correlation and anticorrelation. In a longitudinal study in our laboratory Joss Smith (Smith *et al.* 1988; Smith 1989) tested the same infants on alternate weeks with the VEP and FPL methods. There was a strong

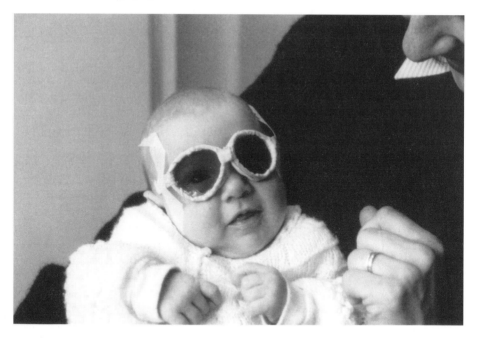

Fig. 6.10(a)

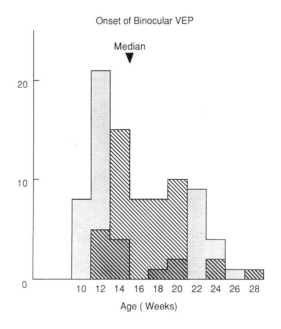

Fig. 6.10(b)

Fig. 6.10 (a) Infant wearing red/green goggles, ready to view the red/green dynamic stereogram. (b) Longitudinal data across a large group of infants (*n* = 104) showing onset of sensitivity to binocularity from both FPL and VEP methods.

correlation between the ages at which a statistically reliable response of each kind was detected, with the average age of onset being about 2 weeks later on the FPL method compared with VEP (Fig. 6.11).

Strictly, positive performance on the correlogram test is not a demonstration of stereopsis. Stereopsis requires the ability not just to distinguish correlation from non-correlation, but to distinguish correlation at different disparities. However, Smith's longitudinal study also tested infants with two different displays: the correlogram stimulus described above and a stereo display in which the background was correlated and a pattern of 42 min arc disparate checks periodically appeared and disappeared. On both VEP and FPL measures, the onset of a response to stereo disparity averaged within a few days of the onset of the correlogram response in the same individual infants, suggesting that a common mechanism underlies both responses (see Fig. 6.12).

Other groups (Fox *et al.* 1980; Held *et al.* 1980; Birch *et al.* 1982; Birch 1993) have concentrated on stereopsis rather than binocular correlation. Birch *et al.*'s measurements use a FPL method with line stereograms rather than random dots; they found that infants will show a preference for a display of three vertical bars in which the central bar has a crossed disparity relative to the others, compared with a set of bars which lie in a single stereo plane. Despite the difference in stimuli, the onset age for disparity sensitivity (typically 12–16 weeks) was close to that found with random-dot displays.

From all these studies, using different behavioural and electrophysiological methods, it is possible to present a fairly clear and well agreed picture which is that sensitivity to binocular disparity begins in human infants at about 3–4 months of age. This means that by about 4 months, postnatally, there must be some mechanism

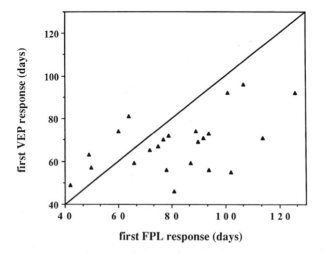

Fig. 6.11 Comparison between the first recorded binocular VEP and first binocular FPL response in infants tested longitudinally.

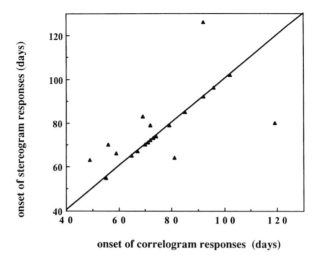

Fig. 6.12 Comparison of the correlogram response and the stereogram response for individual infants.

which is functional within the human visual cortex for signalling binocular interactions. However, there is considerable real individual variation from infant to infant within the range of at least 8–20 weeks (Braddick *et al.* 1983; Wattam-Bell *et al.* 1987). Birch *et al.* (1982) have used their method to test the minimum disparity for which infants show a preference. Their results suggest that after the initial onset of sensitivity, the measure of stereoacuity shows a very rapid increase, typically going from 80 to 1 min arc in a matter of 4–6 weeks.

Stereoacuity can also be called D_{min} i.e. the minimum disparity which can be detected. Equally important in understanding binocular function, is the maximum disparity for which binocular correlation can be detected, called D_{max}. John Wattam-Bell in our team has tested this through infants' preference for a pattern containing bands of high-disparity random dots on a background of uncorrelated dots (Wattam-Bell 1995). This D_{max} measure approximately doubles between 16 and 22 weeks of age. Thus the range of infants' disparity sensitivity expands at both its upper and lower limits, although the increase Wattam-Bell finds for D_{max} is much more gradual than that reported for D_{min} or stereoacuity.

6.5 EYE ALIGNMENT

One possibility is that central mechanisms for binocularity may be mature at an early age but may not be able to function because the infant's eyes are initially poorly aligned. This means that the onset of functional binocularity is dependent on the age of good eye alignment.

A general finding is that a substantial proportion of newborns' eyes are reasonably well aligned and move synchronously. This proportion increases with age. Although there have been reports that large exotropias are common in newborns (Archer 1993), these observations have been criticized as inadequately controlled for versional eye movements and for the large angle alpha (the angle between the visual axis and optical axis of the eye) of newborn infants (Hainline and Riddell 1995, 1996). Furthermore, appropriate changes of vergence for target distance are observed in the majority of infants before 12 weeks of age (see for example Aslin 1993; Hainline and Riddell 1995, 1996). Thus many if not most infants meet the alignment requirements for binocularity before the age at which binocular discriminations can be demonstrated. Further evidence for onset of binocular function being independent of eye alignment comes from studies of Birch and Stager (1985; Birch 1993). They carried out longitudinal FPL stereo tests with strabismic infants, wearing prisms to compensate for the angle of deviation, and found that up to 4 months, the proportion of esotropic infants showing disparity sensitivity was similar to that of a normal group. However, beyond this age, the number giving positive results increased in the normal group but steeply declined among the esotropes. In other words, even when vergence errors were corrected optically in the esotropes, the emergence of disparity sensitivity was still about 4 months. However, later development of these esotropes did show the effects of abnormal vergence. Thus aligned binocular input was necessary to sustain binocular mechanisms in this group even though it was not necessary for their initial development.

Additional evidence that accurate vergence is not the limiting factor comes from a study by Birch *et al.* (1983). They used a periodic version of a three-bar stimulus to generate the same pattern of disparity differences for stereopsis over a wide range of vergence behaviour by the infant. FPL testing with this display gave a similar distribution of onset age for stereopsis as with the usual version.

In summary, it seems that the limiting factor in onset of sensitivity to binocular disparity is unlikely to be at the motor end in terms of alignment. The plasticity of the binocular system will be discussed further in Chapter 9.

6.6 PERCEPTION OF DEPTH AND DISTANCE USING DISPARITY DISCRIMINATION

Of course, these demonstrations really only show that infants can detect disparity differences using cortical modules consisting of populations of cells with differential sensitivity to disparity. It does not tell us whether infants experience stereoscopic depth and whether they use this information to guide actions. Several experiments support the idea that infants experience depth. Held *et al.* (1980) found that infants who showed clear preferences for vertical line patterns containing horizontal disparity did not show a clear preference when the stimulus was rotated through 90° (which appears rivalrous to adults). Granrud (1986) showed that infants who were sensitive to binocular disparity reached more often to the closer of two objects than infants who were insensitive to disparity. Thirdly Yonas *et al.* (1987) showed that infants who had already developed a sensitivity to disparity, considered an object to be the same if it was specified by binocular disparity and by kinetic information. Of course the latter result could be interpreted as considering the match carried out by the same cortical circuits, with no concern for maintaining the specifying information. Chapter 8 considers the development of various action streams linked to selective attention and discusses a study where it is shown that the kinematics of reaching are modified by the infants' use of stereoscopic information (Braddick *et al*. 1996*a*). The results of this study would seem to be additional evidence that sensitivity to disparity is very useful information gained by the 4–5 month old to use in developing accurate reaching and grasping.

6.7 THEORIES OF CORTICAL ORGANIZATION BEFORE AND AFTER THE ONSET OF FUNCTIONAL BINOCULARITY

Anatomically, fibres carrying signals from both eyes have established terminations in the striate cortex well before birth (Rakic 1977), but their separation into ocular dominance columns is not complete for some weeks postnatally (Hubel and Wiesel 1977; Horton and Hedley-White 1984). If the fibres make cortical connections but do not provide the basis for binocular interaction, how are their binocular relationships organized before the onset of stereopsis? A simple hypothesis might be that individual cortical cells do not combine signals from the two eyes. There appears to be little direct evidence on this point from primate developmental physiology. However, in the young kitten (LeVay *et al*. 1978) the evidence is against this idea: before the segregation of ocular dominance columns, many layer IV cells are binocular, unlike those in the adult. Held (1993) proposes that such convergence characterizes an initial state of 'primitive binocularity' in which the two eyes' inputs are simply summed at the earliest cortical stage. On this view, development of disparity sensitivity depends on separating left- and right-eye signals in layer IV, so that they can come to interact in a range of disparity-specific neurons in the upper cortical layers.

However, it is difficult to see how 'primitive binocularity' can be reconciled with the development of sensitivity to random-dot correlograms. A system of neurons which summed signals from the two eyes would be very strongly stimulated by the transitions between anticorrelated and correlated dots, which would resemble transitions between high- and low-contrast dots. Indeed, this is exactly the appearance if presentation of the dot patterns is not separated between the eyes, a condition which elicits strong VEPs in pre-stereoscopic infants (Braddick *et al*. 1980, 1983). Thus it might be expected that correlogram responses, behavioural and VEP, would be observed in the *primitive binocularity* stage, with disparity-sensitive responses appearing later. In direct comparison this dissociation was not found, and sensitivity to correlograms has been seen at much the same age as to stereograms in individual infants. Perhaps binocular inputs are combined in the pre-stereoscopic infant, but in a way which is not spatially specific in the way that would be required for point-by-point summation. At present, the existence and nature of pre-stereoscopic binocularity remains unclear.

Another puzzle is the fact that infants before 3 months can maintain eye alignment and adjust it to converge on a near target. What signal are they using to achieve alignment? In the adult system, a disparity signal provides the main input to achieve this, but these infants are insensitive to disparity. Held (1993) suggests that maximization of the signal in primitive binocular summing neurons might guide vergence; but this is exactly the signal which, as discussed above, we might expect to see in the correlogram VEP and do not find in infants under 4 months of age. Alternatively, if separate monocular signals are available in the visual system of the pre-stereoscopic infant, foveal fixation of a target might be controlled for each eye separately, leading secondarily to binocular alignment. Given the importance of the superior colliculus in guiding fixation, this might be somewhat distinct from the issue of whether monocular signals are separate in the visual cortex. Finally, it has been suggested that accommodative vergence (Judge 1996) may contribute to infants' vergence control. Aslin and Jackson (1979) showed that accommodative demand could drive vergence changes in infants as young as 2 months. However, it seems unlikely that signals related to accommodation could provide the accuracy needed to maintain eye alignment; and if it were supposed to be the main source of early vergence control, it raises a puzzling question of how accommodation–vergence relationships came to be calibrated in the first place.

Another theoretical question is 'What underlies the increase in stereoacuity and D_{max}?' Of these, D_{max} is the easier to understand, at least speculatively. Disparity

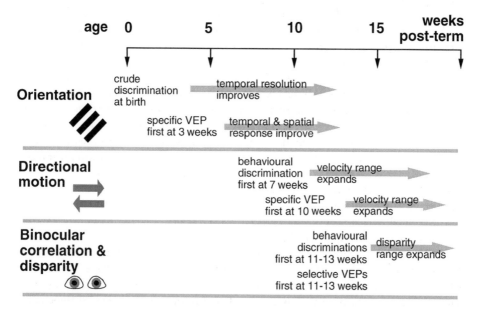

Fig. 6.13 Schematic showing progressive onset of sensitivity for relative orientation, direction, and disparity.

detection requires the interaction of signals from neighbouring points in the combined topographic representation of the binocular field of view. It is reasonable to imagine progressive growth of the lateral intracortical connections serving this interaction. The parallel developmental increases in D_{max} for stereopsis and for motion detection (Wattam-Bell 1995) suggest that a general pattern of extending connections might be responsible for both.

However, stereoacuity has been reported to increase at a much more rapid pace than D_{max}. This increase is also many times faster than the increase of resolution acuity with age, and faster than the increase in vernier acuity (which itself outpaces the increase in resolution acuity; Shimojo *et al.* 1984). There are several possibilities to explain this rapid development of stereoacuity. There could be a range of fine-tuned disparity detectors arising in the cortex, by a developmental process specific to disparity, at a remarkable pace; or, the complete range is established all together at the onset of stereopsis, and the infant takes a comparatively short time to organize and interpret their patterns of output. Neither of these possibilities seem very plausible at present and so it seems that we have no good explanation for why stereoacuity should be so good so early in young infants' lives. Of course in terms of ecological necessity it seems plausible that our evolutionary ancestors would need good stereoacuity at a very young age to ensure survival in an environment where tree to tree swinging was part of everyday life. However, the precise course of development for this highly tuned disparity system is still largely undecided.

6.8 CONCLUSIONS ON EARLY CORTICAL DEVELOPMENT

In conclusion, it seems that populations of cortical neurons in at least V1, V2, and V3 become operational and function to underpin some of the visual discriminations seen in infants in the first few months of life. Figure 6.13 shows a global schematic for the development of specialized channels for orientation, directional motion, and binocularity. The systems underpinning orientation and colour discrimination would seem to operate somewhat earlier than those for relative motion and disparity detection. This might be taken to suggest that at least some aspects of a parvocellular-based system may mature prior to the magnocellular-based system (as suggested in Atkinson 1992). Just as plausibly, it could be that there is different maturation in interconnections between cortical areas and this causes different levels of functioning and different time courses. For example, in terms of directional motion analysis, directionality in V1 responses could be fully mature, but the connections to the response system, enabling a differential response to a stimulus containing two different directions of motion, rather than one, may not be functional. Yet another possibility is that inhibitory mechanisms from higher cortical areas do not inhibit subcortically controlled OKN systems, which give automatic simple responses to unilateral motion. As yet there are many possibilities concerning early plasticity. In Chapter 7 the beginnings of object perception are considered, in which the simpler mechanisms of orientation, relative motion, and colour discrimination in various depth planes must be appropriately combined.

7 Development of integration ('binding') and segmentation processes leading to object perception

Chapter 6 considered the systems responsible for discriminating orientation, colour, motion, and depth in the visual scene were considered. The next stage to consider is combining the outputs of multiple units, to give the infant the perception of surfaces and objects, rather than isolated elements. No attempt is made here to give a full account of development of object perception in infants, as this would take up an entire book in itself. Rather, the initial processes of object segmentation are emphasized and the more cognitive aspects of object categorization are left to other authors who have concentrated their research in these areas (see, for example, the work of Al Yonas, Susan Carey, Elizabeth Spelke, Phillip Kellman, Rene Baillargeon, and Scott Johnson).

Objects are the units by which we divide physical space. They are contrasted with extended surfaces or backgrounds. A fundamental process which takes place in perception is that objects must be separated from their background and then from one another. There is much debate in adult vision about the processes of segmentation (where one object is separated from another) and binding (where common features are locked together within one object). Really these can be two ways of describing the same process.

In J. J. Gibson's (1950) extensive theoretical accounts of spatial perception, he describes objects as physical units that are restricted in terms of spatial extent, temporal duration, and coherence relative to physical forces. Some have argued that what is described as an object depends on the visuocognitive processing of the observer. For example, the planet Earth when viewed from a great distance appears as a round object although in real life the Earth seems to us as an extended surface. It can be argued that as adults, although our viewing distance varies, we have a fixed representation of what are objects in everyday perception and what are surfaces. In some sense, although when we view the floor inside an aeroplane it is viewed as a surface, we have simultaneous knowledge that it is part of a large object (the aeroplane), but we also know it is not a manipulable object. For the purposes of performing successful actions upon objects we need to know how to divide an object from its background, the exact position of its edges (i.e. its size) and the properties of its surfaces (e.g. whether its surfaces are rough or smooth). A primary process in object perception is, therefore, edge detection which can be considered as a basic figure ground process and has been called 'segmentation' by many researchers.

Segmentation or *edge detection* is based on detecting discontinuities within the optical information in the stimulus. As objects tend to be made of particular substances with certain surface properties such as colour, texture, and brightness we can use discontinuities within these attributes to divide one object from another. Of course, in everyday vision not all discontinuities of luminance and texture correspond to separate objects. Shadows or changes of texture on a surface, for example, are marked discontinuities, and if incorrectly interpreted could lead us to assign boundaries between objects incorrectly. To disambiguate such displays we use discontinuities in motion and in depth to separate one object from another, ignoring the obvious discontinuities on particular surfaces.

In real visual scenes most objects are partially occluded by other objects. Often object boundaries traverse areas which are identical in luminance and so to understand that these are a number of complete objects we must fill in the contours where they are occluded. These have been called *illusory contours*. There has been extensive modelling in the literature on adult vision to decide how the visual system produces perception of real and illusory contours (e.g. Marr 1982; Grossberg and Mingolla 1985; Shapley and Gordon 1985). In Marr's model these subjective contours cannot be accounted for by totally linear spatial theory modelling, such as has been suggested for cortical neurons in V1. Rather a preceding non-linear process of rectification is introduced. Responses of this kind have been found in V2 to luminance defined and line terminator defined lines (von der Heydt *et al.* 1984; von der Heydt and Peterhans 1989), although similar responses have also been found in V1 cells (Grosof *et al.* 1993). Models for such non-linear contour responses are similar to those for second order motion (e.g. Wilson *et al.* 1992; Shapley 1994).

The processes whereby objects are perceived as a unit, called object unity, have already been extensively discussed by Gestalt psychologists many years ago in their principles of perception (e.g. Wertheimer 1923; Koffka 1935). The role of motion was expressed as the principle of common fate. The principle of good continuation holds that in general straight or smoothly bending contours usually form the boundaries of units, and the principle of good form states that objects or surfaces are part of one unit if they are similar or grouped. These principles have been explicitly applied to the problem of occlusion by Michotte *et al.* (1964). However, the Gestalt principles do not allow precise quantification of the use of different visual attributes to assign surfaces and objects.

We have looked at development of some very basic segmentation processes using different visual attributes, necessary for separating one object from another and for combining objects into complex spatial arrays by measuring which discontinuities infants can detect and use as they mature. These are described below. Others such as Spelke and Kellman have used a Gibsonian approach to gauge the processes of common motion used by infants in the detection of illusory contours to provide object unity; a good review of this work can be found in Kellman and Arterberry's (1998) chapter on object perception in their recent book. According to the models they propose, unit formation is governed by two separate processes, 'edge-insensitive' and 'edge-sensitive'. The former process utilizes common motion to define an edge but does not require edge relationships (straightness and smoothness of curvature) to perceive the unit. Edge-sensitive processing requires an understanding of hidden boundaries and can be applied in static or dynamic displays. From studies on infants (e.g. Johnson 1998) it would seem that the 'common movement' process is operational before 6 months of age whereas the edge-sensitive processes require appropriate learning and become operational later than 6 months of age. This theoretical divide, into edge-sensitive and edge-insensitive processes, has a certain similarity to the theoretical proposals of Slater *et al.* (1988) and Yonas *et al.* (1987). They have argued that in terms of development there is perceptual analysis of kinetic monocular depth cues in the first few months of life, whereas cues specified by pictorial depth, such as relative size and occlusion (specified by static cues), are not understood and interpreted correctly by infants until after 7 months of age.

One problem in all of these theoretical accounts, may be in separating the parameters of the cues themselves from the processes involved in gauging the attentional salience of the cues to the infant. It may be that the same mechanisms underpin development of both cue discrimination and selective attention, and if this is the case, if the attentional salience scale of the infant changes during development with increasing age, then there will be an apparent parallel change in the infant's understanding of object unity. If certain cues are high on the attentional salience scale at a particular age, due to maturation of a particular mechanism for perceiving unity at this age, then it is difficult to decide which process became functional first and which was a consequence of the maturation of the other.

For this reason, in my theoretical model in Chapter 3, development of the processes involved in attribute binding, object recognition (which includes a notion of the unity and separation of objects from one another), and development of the attentional eye/head movements systems, has been placed at much the same level of development (they may possibly develop as one process). This is to make it clear that at present we do not know whether one of these systems precedes another in functional development, or whether there can be isolated development of one system without contiguous development of another. Further research is needed to separate these possibilities.

7.1 DEVELOPMENT OF SEGMENTATION PROCESSES

Julesz (1981) has proposed a theory of pre-attentive processing, defining classes of local features called 'textons' (such as edge segments and edge terminators), which enable the rapid discrimination of one texture from another for segmenting between objects. Textons embody local phase relationships, i.e. the relative phase of the spatial frequency components making up the pattern elements. Relative phase information, together with amplitude or intensity, will enable a complete specification of any pattern. Certain phase relationships will be 'special' in that they correspond to physical features of the outside world, e.g. the 'peaks-subtract' phase relationship specifies a sharp square-wave edge. Many models of relative phase discrimination propose perception of configuration to be dependent on comparator detectors across spatial frequency channels. Such phase selectivity might, for example, be embodied in channels having even- and odd-symmetric receptive fields, and such mechanisms are known to exist in the cortex rather than subcortex.

Applying these models of adult vision, tests of relative phase and texton discrimination have been used to infer cortical functioning in young infants. It appears that

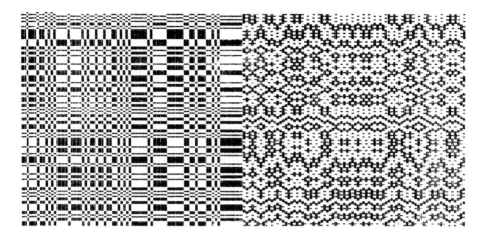

Fig. 7.1 Examples of the texton patterns used to measure segmentation processes in young infants.

1 month olds are insensitive to changes in relative phase, when viewing complex gratings made up of several superimposed spatial frequencies (Braddick *et al.* 1986*b*). Nor do they discriminate between texture patterns shown in Figure 7.1, differing in the type of texton detectors proposed for adults (Atkinson *et al.* 1986*a*). As 3 month olds have no difficulty with such discriminations, we can infer that these cortical mechanisms to allow segmentation to take place come on line between 1 and 3 months of age.

7.2 SEGMENTATION ON THE BASIS OF ORIENTATION

One might imagine that an even simpler form of texture segmentation would be based on merely recognizing areas containing identical single features, such as an area composed of similarly oriented short line segments. This segmentation process would take place after primary visual mechanisms have registered the simple stimulus properties of orientation, and would be used to define distinct surfaces, objects, and events in the visual world. In adults, the presence of orientation differences between line or edge segments making up two textures is very effective in determining visual segmentation (Beck 1966; Olson and Attneave 1970; Nothdurft 1990). Several models of cortical mechanisms responsible for these pre-attentive processes have been proposed (e.g. Sagi and Julesz 1985; Nothdurft 1990). Their principal component is a set of local differencing operations, acting on the output of neurons which are visual filters for specific properties. The differencing function may depend on connections within the cortex providing mutual inhibition between pools of neurons specifying differing orientations.

  We have evidence for these cortical inhibitory mechanisms in infants older than 4 months of age, from measuring their ability to orient towards a rectangular area in the visual field, whose boundary is defined by a change in orientation of the line segments making up the display.

Using forced-choice preferential looking we have measured the infant's ability to detect the change of orientation within the rectangular patch compared with the background which was arranged either to the left or the right of central fixation (see Fig. 7.2). No clear preferential looking for the segmented region is seen in infants younger than 4 months of age, and even at this age the response appears relatively weak (Atkinson and Braddick 1993). Similar paradigms have been used in Ruxandra Sireteanu's research group (Sireteanu and Rieth 1992; Rieth and Sireteanu 1994) who find no evidence for segmentation on the basis of orientation until about 6 months of age. This relatively late onset of ability to segment on the basis of orientation suggests that other mechanisms for segmenting and localizing objects in the visual world, such as contrast cues and differential motion, may be more robust and useful in the first few months of life. Of course it may be that even in adult vision, the primary segmenting mechanisms use crude intensity differences to parse the visual scene and that these decisions are then confirmed by additional information provided by elaborate texture and phase comparators. It may also be that the orienting mechanism necessary for rapid detection of objects in the peripheral field does not use information processed in the cortex very effectively, but relies instead on crude information provided by subcortical systems including the superior colliculus.

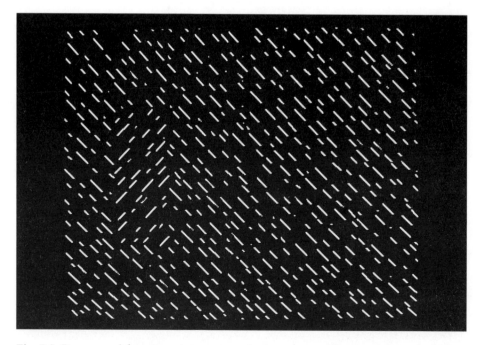

Fig. 7.2 Pattern used for orientation segmentation experiment. The experimenter looks for a preferential look to the side of the display containing the differently oriented patch.

7.3 SEGMENTATION ON THE BASIS OF MOTION

In Chapter 6 the initial stages of segmentation on the basis of relative motion in young infants have already been discussed. Much of this discussion could have formed the beginning of this section on segmentation on the basis of motion. Here, this discussion is taken a stage further, to discuss detection of coherent motion in a background of incoherent motion.

There have been many studies of adults' ability to detect motion coherence—i.e., the coherent direction of movement of a percentage of the dots in a field of randomly moving dots (Newsome and Pare 1988; Scase *et al.* 1996). The percentage required to be coherently moving to allow threshold detection of coherence is called the 'coherence threshold'. To process this display, seen in Fig. 7.3, local and global processing must take place over extended regions of the visual field, so that within one region of visual space random movements of some of the dots must be ignored and others with common movement must be amalgamated into a bounded region.

There has been extensive research using functional magnetic resonance imaging (fMRI), pioneered by Zeki's and Tootell's groups (Watson *et al.* 1993; Tootell *et al.*

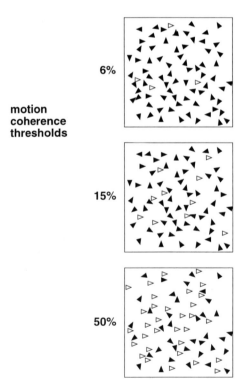

motion coherence thresholds

6%

15%

50%

Fig. 7.3 Motion coherence schematic. The percentage of coherently moving dots which allows discrimination of direction of motion is called the motion coherence threshold.

1995) looking at human cortical motion processing comparing static and moving stimuli. Figure 7.4 is an example of one of the images from our own fMRI studies (Braddick *et al*. 1998*a*), where we have been specifically interested in the systems in the brain which are not only specific for moving stimuli over static, but must be involved in processing coherent movement over relatively large regions of space.

Figure 7.4 shows the regions of the adult cortex, notably V5 and V3a, which are differentially more active when movement is coherent compared with when it is present but randomly incoherent. Interestingly, V1, primary visual cortex, seems to show larger activation for incoherent random motion than for coherent motion.

7.4 INCREASED SENSITIVITY TO COHERENT MOTION WITH AGE

It was discussed in Chapter 6 how sensitivity to relative motion, allowing segmentation, develops rapidly in the first few months of life. We can also gain a picture of global integrative motion processes by measuring coherence thresholds in infancy (Wattam-Bell 1994). We do not yet have comprehensive data on how coherence sensitivity increases from infancy to adult vision. However, we know about a point in between in childhood from studies recently carried out on normal 4–8 year olds and on children with the same mental age who have Williams syndrome (Atkinson *et al*. 1999). Because of our interest in the split between dorsal and ventral stream development, the children's motion coherence thresholds have been compared with their thresholds in a form coherence task (see Fig. 7.5).

Figure 7.6 shows the relative improvement of form and motion coherence thresholds with age. An important point to note is that, although both are relatively mature by 8 years of age, form coherence thresholds are adult-like much earlier than those for motion coherence. These differences between form and motion coherence will be considered when plasticity is discussed in Chapter 9.

7.5 SEGMENTATION BY LINE TERMINATORS

The idea of 'illusory contours' has already been briefly described above. Will Curran in our group has recently carried out a series of experiments measuring infants' ability to detect such illusory contours using line terminators. From previous studies (e.g. Trieber and Wilcox. 1980; Ghim 1990; Reith and Sireteanu 1993) there is the suggestion that this ability develops before 6 months of age, but for many of the studies the stimuli used allow the infant to detect the contour using an alternative mechanism to one for detecting line terminators. Curran *et al*. (1999) have tested 2–4 month olds using a preferential looking paradigm where one of the stimuli contained a moving illusory contour made up of abutting lines, and the other pattern had the same number of terminators, which were overlapping and not aligned (see Fig. 7.7).

The stimuli were dynamic so that a smoothly moving illusory line oscillated back

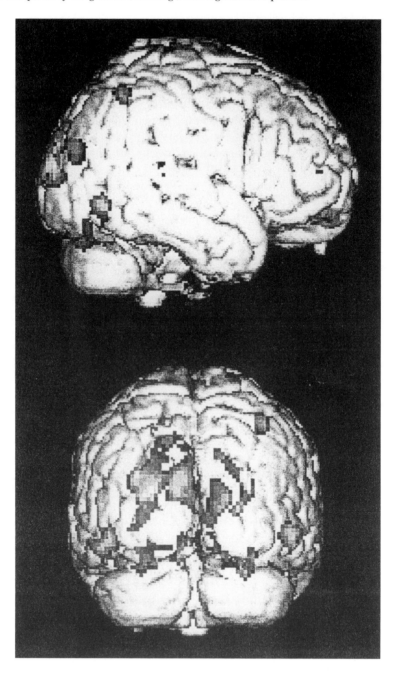

Fig. 7.4 Functional magnetic resonance imaging image from an adult, showing areas V5 and V3A which are specifically involved in processing coherent rather than random motion.

and forth on one side of the display, while the other side showed overlapping lines oscillating in synchrony. The impression of the illusory contour was much more compelling in the moving sequence than when stationary. It was found that there was a preference for the illusory contour in the infants older than 12 weeks but not in 8 week olds, if the velocity used was 6.6 degree/s. If, however, the motion was speeded up to 9.5 degree/s it is possible to see the preference for the illusory contour even in the younger infants of 8 weeks. The change in velocity tuning with age for young infants, as their motion detecting systems develop, has already been discussed in Chapter 6. It was found that 8–12 week olds showed directional responses for velocities between 7 and 14 degree/s, but not for faster and slower speeds outside this range. In the experiment with moving illusory contours, we are possibly tapping a process which combines information from both the ventral (V2—line terminator detection) and dorsal (relative movement detection) streams, and the response of the infant is decided by the relative stage of development for these two mechanisms and their interactions between them. In neuroanatomy, Shipp and Zeki (1989) found that whereas ascending projections from V2 to V5 go exclusively from the thick stripes of V2 (part of the dorsal stream), the descending projections infiltrate the thin stripes and interstripes. For infants to respond to line terminators their visual system would need to register the continued alignment of the inducing line terminators and this may be the role of the ascending and descending projections between V2 and V5, which are already starting to function at 2 months of age. This can be compared with the results on motion-based segmentation discussed in the previous chapter (Wattam-Bell 1996*a*,*d*), suggesting that a number of these integrative processes take off in development at about the same time. As these processes are likely to depend on

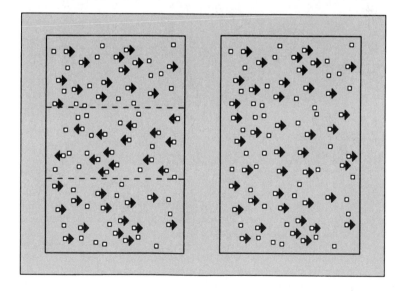

Fig. 7.5(a) (See next page for caption.)

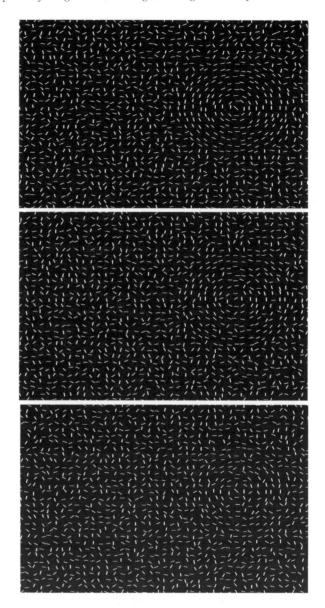

Fig. 7.5(b)

Fig. 7.5 (a) Motion coherence stimulus. The child has to identify the region of dots moving differently from the rest of the display. The threshold is found when coherence is reduced by a proportion of flickering dynamic noise dots. The child is asked to put their hand on 'the road in the snowstorm'. (b) Form coherence stimulus for three different levels of coherence. The child has to identify the region where line segments are arranged in circles (randomly orientated segments elsewhere). The threshold is found when coherence is reduced by a proportion of randomly orientated lines. The child is asked to put their hand on 'the ball in the grass'.

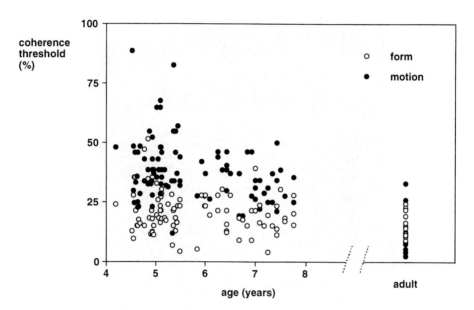

Fig. 7.6 Changes in motion and form coherence thresholds with age. Each dot represents the threshold for an individual child.

feedback mechanisms from extrastriate areas to striate, it seems that even if the ascending pathways to visual cortex are starting to operate shortly after birth, these integrative mechanisms require an extra month or so of experience to co-ordinate different areas within the cortical circuits.

7.6 OBJECT RECOGNITION FROM BIOLOGICAL MOTION

Chapter 6 has already discussed how one surface or object can be segregated from another using relative motion or relative disparity information. So far we have always been talking about rigid surfaces. However, many important objects in the infant's world are non-rigid, for example movements of the hand and arm, facial expressions, and whole body movements. Of course, the task for the visual system in analysing the shape of non-rigid objects is more complicated than the same analysis for rigid objects. Many theorists have tackled this problem of transformation from optical properties of non-rigid motion to the deduction of objects' shapes in adult vision (e.g. Johansson 1975; Cutting 1986) and there have been a number of studies on infants' perception of non-rigid forms. Bertenthal and Proffitt and their colleagues are the main group who have investigated infants' understanding of biological motion (see Bertenthal 1993 for a summary). When 3 and 5 month olds were habituated to a Johansson light display sequence of an upright walking person they showed dishabituation to a sequence of the images when inverted (Bertenthal *et al.* 1987).

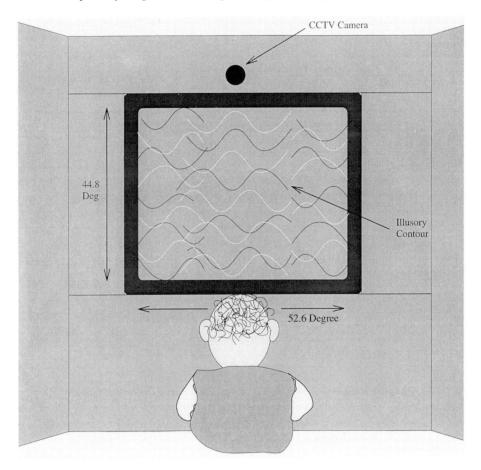

Fig. 7.7 Schematic of the pattern used for measuring dynamic illusory contours in infants.

With static snapshots from the same sequence, the dishabituation did not occur. However, this result in itself does not necessarily imply that the infant perceives a person walking in either the inverted or upright display. Further evidence from the same group does imply that by 5 months of age the infant infers that it is a person walking in the upright light displays. These studies used *phase shifting* (varying the starting locations in the periodic motions of particular point lights) to degrade the percept of a walking person. Bennett Bertenthal and his colleagues found that both 3 and 5 month olds discriminate normal from phase shifted upright displays. When inverted, only the 3 month olds discriminated the displays. An inference from this study might be that the superior discrimination using phase information with upright displays due to the fact that upright displays are perceived as more than an interesting display of lights by older infants (over 5 months) and are seen as a moving person, with the percept being disrupted by phase shifting. As the inverted displays are not perceived as a person walking, the correct phase relationships are not critical and salient for discrimination. This result would suggest that infants need to be at least 5 months of age before they use phase information to infer the concept of a moving person from the light displays. Before this age they discriminate between different phase relations but do not use the information to categorize the displays into objects. The discrimination of spatial phase relations to enable discrimination of rigid static displays by 3 months of age, has already been discussed in our own studies. These results for the discrimination of phase agree well with the time course found for temporal phase manipulations in studies by Bertenthal's group (Bertenthal 1993). The difference would seem to be that the perception of objects, beyond the first stage which is the segmentation of edges, may be delayed in terms of development for non-rigid displays until at least 5 months of age. Again evidence can be seen for later development in the use of dynamic relative motion cues compared with static cues. This could be taken as evidence of later development in the cortical underpinnings for relative motion, including biological motion—dorsal stream areas such as V5 and MST—(Middle Superior Temporal) than for the (ventral stream) systems which may underpin recognition of static objects.

7.7 SPATIAL GROUPING ABILITY

Segmenting one part of visual space from another to discern separate objects is a starting point for understanding the layout of visual space. The developing child needs not only to be able to separate one object from another, but also to understand the spatial relationships between objects. Although clearly even newborn infants have a crude sense of spatial layout in that they can coarsely localize objects in space, they do not possess the ability to understand detailed spatial relationships until relatively late in infancy.

One method used for gauging deficits of spatial cognition in adult patients is the copying of block designs. Results from many studies using such tests have shown disorders of spatial analytic functioning in patients with specific focal lesions. Differences have been suggested for patients with left and right hemisphere lesions. Patients with left damage tend to oversimplify and omit detail, while right posterior lesions cause difficulties with the overall global configuration. Similar differences have been found in children with left and right focal lesions (Stiles-Davis *et al.* 1985; Stiles and Nass 1991). It appears that in spontaneous construction with bricks young children progress through a series of stages (see examples of these stages in Fig. 7.8).

Here it can be seen that simple spatial stacking strategies characterize the designs of 18 month olds, whereas by 3 years elaborate multiple constructions are generated, showing rudimentary understanding of a variety of spatial relationships ('on', 'inside', 'next to', 'parallel to', 'joined to'). In collaboration with Joan Stiles, we have been designing constructional tasks, involving copying block designs containing different spatial relationships, appropriate to the copying abilities of children of different ages. Eventually it is hoped to have an understanding of the constraints of the infant's understanding of grouping and segmentation, from the start of reaching at 6 months of age through childhood. At present some data are available on early reaching (see Chapter 8) and on the constructions made by infants from 12 months of age to 5 years of age. It is almost impossible to persuade a 1 year old to construct anything but an isolated stack of one or two bricks and this is what they spontaneously

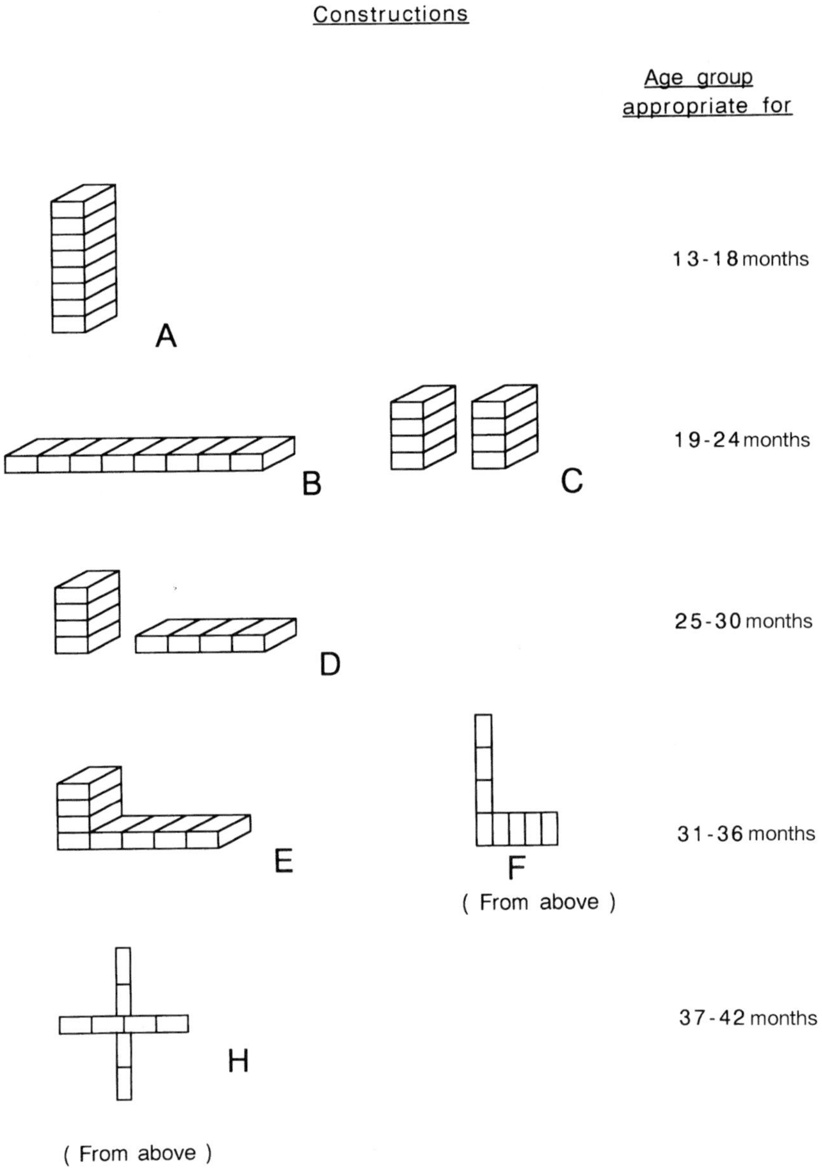

Constructions

Age group
appropriate for

A

13-18 months

B

C

19-24 months

D

25-30 months

E

F

(From above)

31-36 months

H

(From above)

37-42 months

Fig. 7.8(a) (See opposite page for caption.)

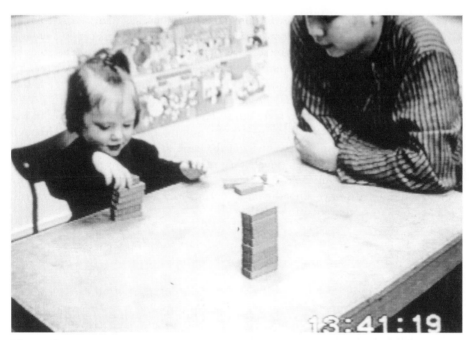

Fig. 7.8(b)

Fig. 7.8 (a) Sequence of block constructions spontaneously made by children between 18 months and 4 years. The complexity of the construction increases with age, as does the complexity of the construction that the child is able to copy. (b) Child copying a block construction of a stack.

start to make from 9 to 18 months of age. Even taking into account their somewhat limited motoric skills and their love of demolition, this result suggests that their extreme focal attention to one point in space at a time, represents a deficit in global attention to the configurational properties of the constructions and a lack of understanding as to how the relative parts of a complex construction fit together to make a global shape. However, it can be seen from studies on orientation and motion segmentation (discussed above) and from other studies of global and local pattern processing in 3–4 month olds (e.g. Ghim and Eimas 1988) that very young infants can, under some circumstances, process both global and local features at the same time, for parsing the visual world. This can perhaps be taken as evidence for a dramatic separation in development between the relatively sophisticated processing in perceptual discriminations in early infancy, and the lack of integration of this perceptual information, with that necessary for planning and guiding actions. Even somewhat older infants of 18 months, who would have no difficulty in discriminating a design made up of a simple stack of bricks from one made up of a line of bricks, fail to be able to copy the latter construction, but have no difficulty in copying a tower of bricks. It seems that construction of 'next-to' relations may require more analysis of the spatial array than a spatially well defined construction involving 'on' or 'in' relations. In stacking, elements in the construction provide support for new items; 'next-to' relations are not defined within a single locus, with new items being placed in any position around other items. As suggested above, infants by 6 months of age seem to be able to apply segmenting principles to separate one object from another. However, spatially representing the global layout of these objects over a relatively large area of visual field requires not only parallel segmentation of multiple objects, but also continuous updating of this map to take into account self-movement and object movement, plus the ability to switch between global and focal representations. Although young infants would seem to have many of the basic mechanisms necessary for spatial representation already operational, they seem to lack much of the integrative information processing which enables those with a mature system to unconsciously represent the visual world, smoothly and continuously and to switch scale at will, back and forwards, from local to global.

7.8 CONCLUSIONS

It seems that in early infancy there are mechanisms operating to allow the child to separate objects and surfaces from one another. Multiple cues to discontinuity and 'edge detection' are available (luminance, colour, relative motion, relative depth), but each of these systems have their own time-scale for functional onset after which they can be used in parallel to discriminate objects from their backgrounds. The ability to switch scale from local features of objects to the overall shape of objects would seem to be more problematical for deciding a functional onset date. There is rather little research on these switching abilities, although recent studies by researchers such as Liz Spelke and Scott Johnson are suggesting that there are certain common principles that are mastered early in infancy and others much later (see, for example, Johnson 1998). An even more elaborate stage of spatial analysis is required for combining perceptual object processing with actions operating on objects. Block design copying tasks have briefly been discussed in this chapter and will be returned to in Chapter 8 on the development of reaching and grasping. There seems to be a split in development between systems operating within the dorsal cortical stream controlling actions and those in the ventral stream controlling perceptual discriminations. Dorsal stream processing for spatial cognition, including actions on objects, matures relatively late compared with ventral stream processing for object discrimination and recognition.

8   The interlinked approach to development of attention and action

8.1   INTRODUCTION

This chapter will consider the development and interlinking of two major systems —first, the attentional system for selecting what to look at and what to reach for, and second, the action systems which can be invoked in these switches. Not all of the attentional systems will be discussed in detail, nor will there be a full description of the development of the kinetics of reaching and grasping. Rather, this discussion will be focused on some recent results with a diverse set of paradigms, to study some aspects of this extremely complicated set of mechanisms. First, what developmentalists mean by infant attention is considered. Then, we consider development of specific systems, both for attention and actions. The remaining loose ends are identified at the chapter's conclusion.

8.2   WHAT DO WE MEAN BY 'ATTENTION'?

For developmentalists, numerous different aspects of behaviour are thought to reflect 'attention' (or the operations of attentional brain mechanisms) in infants and young children. For example, many children with severe neurological deficits are unable to 'fix and follow'. This is the neurologist's terminology, meaning that these children are unable to concentrate their attention ('foveate') on an object and then track it as it moves from their point of fixation. In a somewhat different context children who have been labelled 'hyperactive' have attentional disorders in that they are thought to have 'short attention spans'—meaning that they do not concentrate their attention on the task in hand, but rapidly switch attention from one thing to another, losing concentration very rapidly. These shifts of attention are often accompanied by motor movements. The syndrome known as the attentional deficit hyperactive disorder (ADHD) has become a very popular label for children between the ages of 4 and 10 years, who are very distractible and find it difficult to sustain attention on the task in hand. These children often show other behavioural problems, such as conduct disorder and aggression. There is much debate concerning its diagnosis and treatment. Some neurological syndromes are characterized by attentional disorders such as an inability to switch attention from one level of analysis to another. For example, it has been claimed that children with Williams' syndrome (a rare genetic disorder), are often found to attend to the local parts of a design or pattern without being able to switch to the overall global design (see discussion in Chapter 9).

For developmentalists studying infants and very young pre-school children, improvements in attention span have been regarded as synonymous with improvements in speed of learning or improved information processing. A good example of this is seen in the work of researchers such as Bornstein, Fagan, and Cohen (e.g. Bornstein 1985), where improvements of attentional processing are measured in young infants by measuring the increase in the rate of visual habituation seen over the first few months of life. Using this idea, recent studies of infant visual attention have suggested a relationship between infant attentional capacity and later cognitive capacity. This places 'attention' as the central gate or switch in visual processing. Without attentional control the infant's brain is seen as a passive receiver. Certainly, over the first few months of life, the infant actively starts to select what is scrutinized; this process is tuned up throughout childhood, culminating in the adult's multilevel attentional systems.

8.3 EARLY STAGES OF DEVELOPMENT OF SELECTIVE ATTENTION

In Chapter 3 the various stages of development of visual attentional mechanisms were discussed in outline. The first part of this process was defined as the integration of crude subcortical orienting systems with cortical attentional systems for the control of directed eye and head movements. These processes are developed to enable the infant to switch attention from one object to another, and are therefore presumed to take place either simultaneously with or after segmentation and binding processes. These attentional switches involve a 'disengage' process, to allow the infant to stop attending and processing one object and switch to another.

At a later age attentional mechanisms must develop to allow the infant to decide the target object in reaching and grasping. The attentional mechanisms controlling eye and head movements, already operational, must be integrated with the newly acquired motoric skills in hand manipulation. This process involves the development of near-distance systems for reaching and grasping. The infant develops initially crude arm extension and whole-hand grasp, and these motor systems must take visual information concerning the position of the object in space into account. This will involve discerning, at least, distance information, although initially this could be information from monocular depth cues rather than binocular. The striking relationship between the initial discrimination of stereoscopic depth cues at about 4 months of age with the onset of more accurately directed reaching and grasping a month later suggests that one system is readily linked to the other in the cortex (Braddick *et al.* 1996*a*). There have been suggestions that infants at an early stage of reaching do not always foveate the object which they are reaching for, which might suggest that the integration between eye, head, and hand control systems is not always robust or even necessary for reaching crudely in nearby space. By 6–9 months of age normal infants are compulsive reachers, they reach for anything which is available within arm's length. However, we have found from a number of our recent studies on reaching that after this initial compulsive reaching stage there may be a small reduction in reaching, as the child starts to learn about the 'graspability' of objects. An apparently 'ungraspable' object (such as a large surface or very large object) will not elicit a reach. This suggests that, at the very least, crude object information about the relative size and distance of the object and the size of the infant's hand must be integrated soon after the initiation of motor programs for reaching. At one point in time the infant's perceptual system for object recognition may be more refined and developed than the reaching and grasping action system; this may be indicated by the fact that sophisticated discriminations have been demonstrated in preferential looking in infants at about 3–6 months of age whereas reaching preferences of equivalent complexity are not demonstrated until a later stage.

The various models of visual attention in the adult system were considered briefly in Chapter 3. In the pre-motor theory, selective attention for spatial location or for object recognition involves circuits controlling a number of motor action modules, involved also in object analysis. This pre-motor theory rests on evidence from neurophysiological studies, in which some parietal and frontal areas contain a representation which relates spatial locations, action control and attention, and ablation of these areas causes inattention (neglect) to objects in particular parts of space. Inattention is also accompanied by motor deficits, in particular of movements made to that part of space.

At present we have rather limited knowledge of the developmental time-scale of the various parts of these attention/action circuits in human infants. We can consider the development of attentional and action systems as development of a set of cortical systems, paralleling what we know about the adult systems which are operating. Hence, one way of considering the development of selective attention is to attempt to identify changes in the properties of stimuli that are selected by infants at different ages, to drive their motor actions. We will take this approach in this chapter in considering development of specific action streams.

In considering development of these attention and action systems, when we see either a failure to make an action or an inappropriate action by an infant, it is often difficult to pin-point the neural basis of the limitation. Is it that the infant has not got a well developed attentional system? Is it that the infant cannot segment the objects from their background at this stage of development? Or is it that the infant has not developed adequate motor control to generate the appropriate responses? Nor is it sensible to think of these processes as independent and separable. They are in fact mutually dependent, and involve multiple feedback from one system to another.

8.4 ATTENTION AND ACTION SYSTEMS CONTROLLING HEAD AND EYE MOVEMENTS

8.4.1 Model for improvements in attentional processing early in life

In many of our own studies orienting head and eye movements have been measured as a correlate of the infant's shift of attention from one target to another. In general, the ease of eliciting these eye movements improves with age, particularly if more than one target is in the field of view simultaneously (as is of course the usual situation in everyday vision). In earlier models, I have already suggested that the rapid improvement in the ability to make attentional shifts at about 3 months of age might reflect a changeover from subcortical control to cortical control mechanisms (Atkinson 1984: Braddick and Atkinson 1988). The suggested circuitry for attentional shifts are schematized in Fig. 8.1.

Simple reflex eye movements, controlled by subcortical mechanisms (largely the superior colliculus), seem to be operational from birth, but cortical networks (within the parietal and frontal lobes) are needed to enable older infants to move their eyes rapidly between targets that are competing with one another for the infant's attention. Mark Johnson's (1990) model has also as its core this subcortical/cortical transition in attentional development. However, he attempts to go one stage further by adding the idea of relating changes in oculomotor behaviour to progressive maturation of layers within the primary visual cortex. In this model he suggests that the deeper layers of visual cortex mature before the more superficial ones and that the latter contain inhibitory connections. This developmental sequence may allow certain cortical circuits to become functional before others and certain behavioural correlates to be present before others.

Part of this attentional switching must require the infant to cancel attention to one object and shift it to another. In adult vision, these shifts of attention often coincide with shifts of fixation (foveation). Eye movements made when shifting attention as a response to the sudden appearance of a new visual target are often called 'reflexive' or 'exogenous' because we cannot easily inhibit them and they seem to happen automatically without any planning. Measuring these shifts of gaze, for newly appearing stimuli in the periphery, has been the main way that we have measured

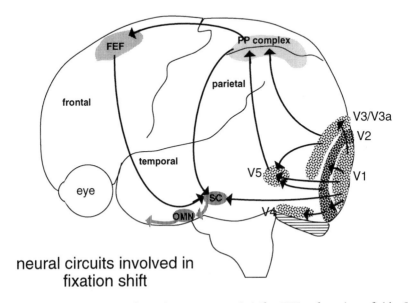

neural circuits involved in
fixation shift

Fig. 8.1 Schematized circuitry for making attentional shifts. FEF = frontal eye fields; SC = superior colliculus; OMN = ocularmotor nuclei; PP = posterior parietal.

improvements in attention with age in infants. Alternatively, eye movements may be made without the sudden appearance of a new stimulus and seem to be driven by an internal searching or scanning process, for a particular part of the object or particular object. These are called 'endogenous', 'intentional', or 'voluntary' in that we assume (at least in adults) some internal goal-oriented mechanism in operation. We can use the changes in scanning eye movements made as the infant grows older as a way of monitoring changes in these endogenous processes. A third possibility is to measure changes in accommodation within the eye as the infant first focuses on one object and then shifts to another object of attention by shifting in the depth plane, either nearer or further away than the first target. It can be assumed that these changes in focusing are associated with internal shifts of attention.

To summarize, three different methods have been used for looking at attentional control of eye movements in infant development.

1. Measurements of orienting to new stimuli in the periphery as seen in saccadic shifts to a peripheral target when an object appears.

2. Measurement of changes in scanning eye movements within the features of an object.

3. Measurements of changes of accommodation for targets at different distances.

8.4.1.1 *Measurements of orienting to new stimuli in the periphery as seen in saccadic shifts to a peripheral target when an object appears*

Both endogenously (internally) controlled and exogenously (externally) controlled overt attentional shifts have been measured in infants by monitoring saccades made from the central field into the peripheral visual field to foveate an object of interest. The spatial limitations of foveation have been called the 'extent of the visual field', and the clinical term for making such measures is 'perimetry'. Effective field size has been found to increase over the first year of life (e.g. Van Hof-van Duin and Mohn 1986; Schwartz *et al.* 1987) and in particular over the first few months.

The newborn or 1 month old's attentional field appears to be relatively limited in lateral extent to about 20–30°, this being the visual angle over which a stimulus can elicit a foveating saccade. There are many early studies measuring attentional fields (e.g. Tronick 1972; Harris and MacFarlane 1974; Aslin and Salapatek 1975; MacFarlane *et al.* 1976; reviewed in Salapatek 1975). Reduced visual fields have been found if a central target remains visible when the peripheral target appears (e.g. Harris and MacFarlane 1974; Aslin and Salapatek 1975; Finlay and Ivinski 1984). However, this effect of a competing central target seems to decrease with age. From this result, it seems likely that as well as increased sensitivity with age, a second process is developing. This process is needed to relinquish attention from the central target and shift attention to the peripheral target. Hence, changes in covert attention have been studied by modifying the simple foveation paradigm to include a distracting or competing stimulus ('probe' or 'mask'), which captures visual attention and prevents or delays saccadic shifts of attention to other targets.

This 'competition effect' where the most recently appearing target has to compete with the already attended target, has been extensively investigated in a series of studies in our own laboratory (Atkinson and Braddick 1985; Braddick and Atkinson 1988; Atkinson *et al*. 1988, 1992, Hood 1993; Atkinson and Hood 1997). Of course, the general apparent increase with age in effective field size could be in part due to increased sensitivity (Atkinson *et al*. 1992). We have attempted to dissociate the effects of improved contrast sensitivity and acuity with age, from improved ability to disengage from a central fixated target and make a saccade to a newly appearing peripheral target. The direction and latency of saccadic eye movements, exogenously triggered by the onset of peripherally located visual targets, were measured. In many of our earlier studies the stimuli used as fixation and orienting targets were relatively large patterned patches consisting of one cycle of square wave grating (12° wide and 32° high, the inner edge being at 23° eccentricity). The mean luminance of these targets was matched to the background. The contrast of the grating could be adjusted either up or down to make the target more or less visible. The observer, who is unaware of the location of the peripheral target, records the direction and time of the first horizontal saccade using a hand-operated switch to give an estimate of the saccadic latency. Using a psychophysical staircase procedure, we estimated the average threshold contrast which reliably produced orienting eye movements to the peripheral target. In these studies we have found that this threshold was about 35% contrast for the 1 month olds and 16% contrast for 3 month olds. Below these thresholds, infants would not refixate the targets with a probability above chance.

The effect of competition from a second identical target remaining in central vision, on the detection rate and latency to refixate a peripheral target was examined, using targets at the thresholds estimated for a non-competition target. Non-competition and competition conditions were examined in the same infants. The latencies of 1 month olds were significantly more affected by competition than 3 month olds. One month olds showed considerable difficulty in disengaging from the central target if it remained visible when the peripheral target appeared. However, because these studies involved equating the two age groups for sensory detectability of the target, we concluded that the remaining significant differences between age groups were due to the additional factor—namely, the 'disengage' mechanism. This finding has been replicated in a study of infants in this age range using rather different targets (Johnson *et al*. 1991). However, in Johnson *et al*.'s study no attempt was made to match the age groups on detection sensitivity, so the competition effect is likely to be due to both differences in sensitivity with age and differences in the ability to disengage. Additional conditions used in our own studies have also shown that in competition the disengage differences between 1 and 3 month olds are also found if two peripheral targets (one on each side of fixation) simultaneously appear. This result further confirms the involvement of a switching mechanism, to enable attention to move from one location to another. However, this need not necessarily be a switch from fovea to periphery; it can also be between two peripheral locations.

In many of our studies using the fixation shift paradigm we have used a display which contains a face-like configuration as the stimulus for initial fixation with the phases reversing bar as the peripheral stimulus (see figure for counterpointing in Chapter 9). We find the same problem of disengagement under the condition of competition, for our very young normally developing infants (under 3 months of age) with this stimulus, with older infants showing slightly longer mean latencies for competition than for non-competition (although this difference does not reach statistical significance for infants over 3 months of age). The mean latencies for individual infants for non-competition and for competition are shown in Fig. 8.2, and these data have been used on normal infants to examine development of attention in various groups of children with neurological problems.

Infants in the first 3 months of life appear to have difficulty in disengaging attention from a foveally viewed target. They appear to sustain attention on the first target which they fixate and do not easily shift their gaze to a newly appearing target. If the length of time for which a stimulus is fixated is a reasonable measure of the length of time for which the infant shows sustained attention then this conclusion does not fit well alongside those who believe that sustained attention improves steadily from birth over the first few months of life, as the infant takes in more and information about the stimulus. We would have to conclude that sustained attention was longer lasting and better in a newborn than a 3–4 month old in the competition condition. How do we then know if the behavioural result of extensive fixation on a single target signifies good sustained attention and information gathering, as has

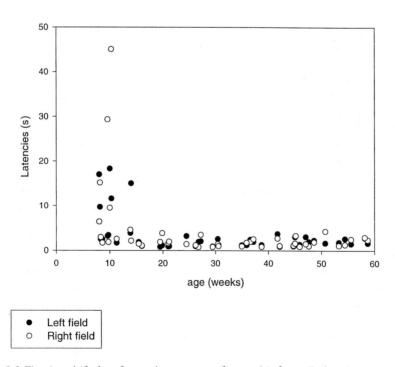

Fig. 8.2 Fixation shift data from a large group of normal infants. Each point represents the mean latency for an individual child. Here the central target was a face-like configuration, rather than a bar pattern.

been argued in 4 month olds, or is it a sign of a problem with disengaging attention from the central stimulus, as we propose in newborns? By monitoring heart rate alongside fixations, John Richards (1989; Richards and Casey 1992) suggests that the problem of disengagement can be separated, from improvements in sustained attention. However, there are few published studies to date where heart rate monitoring alongside eye movement monitoring have been successfully achieved in very young infants (newborns and 1–2 month olds). More data along these lines will need to be collected before we can be sure that lengthy looking times signify increased information processing rather than an inability to disengage looking from one stimulus and shift to another.

Saccadic refixations have also been studied in pre-term infants in comparison with term infants. Foreman *et al.* (1991) compared the latency to refixate with a chequered stimulus and the duration of fixation on that stimulus for term and pre-term groups. Initial fixation time was found to follow a similar developmental function for both infant groups, but an acceleration of development was found for the pre-term group from latency measures over the first 30 postnatal days. This result is similar to a finding from our own studies on healthy very low birth weight pre-term infants (see Chapter 9), who showed shorter latencies at 4–5 weeks post-term than their post-term age-matched control infants, born at term (Atkinson *et al.* 1991).

In a number of our early studies we suggested that there were problems of disengagement not only in very young normal infants but also in older children with neurological impairments. In one of our studies (Hood and Atkinson 1990) we tested a group of neurologically impaired children with the same competition/non-competition fixation shift paradigm as described above. Some of this group of older children showed behaviour similar to the 1 month olds, in that they refixated and appeared to shift attention in non-competition conditions, but failed to refixate if the central stimulus remained visible in competition conditions. However, some of these same children showed a significant visual evoked potential (VEP) to this peripheral target while fixating the central target. This result suggests that the sensory detection mechanism, responsible for generating the VEP, was operating normally, while the attentional disengage processes of attention were not.

We have studied several groups of infants with severe neurological problems including infants who have undergone complete hemispherectomy to relieve intractable focal epilepsy. Study of vision in two of these infants (Braddick *et al.* 1992) provided an opportunity to investigate the activity of the subcortical pathway in isolation from cortical influence, allowing a direct test of the role of cortical mechanisms in the competition effect. Hemispherectomy was carried out on one child at 5 months and the other at 8 months of age. Removal of the cortical hemisphere obliterates the cortical representation of the contralateral visual field. However, as the surgery involves the removal of tissue from above the level of the thalamus, it leaves the retinocollicular pathways intact on both sides of the brain. Both infants were seen pre-operatively and showed very poor visual behaviour, with no consistent shifts of visual attention in informal testing. This was probably in part due to a combination of epilepsy and the heavy medication regimen used to attempt to control their seizures. However, in postoperative testing, both children were visually alert with a full range of eye movements. Both infants had hemiparesis contralateral to the removed hemisphere but were capable of reaching across the midline when they foveated an object of interest. However, this did not occur spontaneously, and each child appeared to ignore completely toys presented in the affected hemifield, although they promptly reached for the same toys in the ipsilateral 'good' half-field. This behaviour is consistent with a loss of visual input from the contralateral visual field.

Each infant was tested on a version of the fixation shift procedure with the central face configuration. The results for one infant are shown at three postoperative sessions in Fig. 8.3. Both infants showed performance considerably above chance in the non-competition condition in orienting to the peripheral target in either half-field. Thus, they could orient to a target which did not have a cortical representation. We explored different aspects of the task with the two children. For one child we tested orienting using each eye alone. She could respond above chance to both the left and right with the right eye (contralateral to the left cortex which had been removed). With the left eye she could only make saccades into the left half field, but not to the right. This result suggests that no uncrossed pathway, capable of transmitting information from the left eye to the damaged left side of the brain, can elicit saccadic eye movements. We tested the other child under competition conditions. He showed reduced saccadic shifts when the peripheral target appeared on his bad side, but rapid shifts into his good field. He often blinked and nodded his head when the target appeared in his bad field, as though to unlock his attention from the central stimulus. One of the infants also showed shorter latencies to respond to the target in his 'good' field (the right) compared with his 'bad' field.

The important finding from this study is to show that both infants are capable of producing saccadic eye movements to stimuli presented in the 'blind' field, which would support the idea that subcortical pathways can subserve this orienting under non-competition conditions. However, cortical control appears to be needed to deal with competing targets (this result is shown in Fig. 8.3. for one of the infants). The behaviour of these infants has some similarity to adult hemispherectomized patients, who can make visual discriminations in the hemianopic visual field, without being consciously aware of the stimuli (Perenin 1978; Perenin and Jeannerod 1978; Ptito *et al.* 1987). Of course, we cannot ask the infants about their visual experience, so we do not know how similar it is to that of adult patients in the absence of striate cortex, which has been described as 'blindsight' (Pöppel *et al.* 1973; Weiskrantz 1986).

The effects of competition between fixation targets has been found in adults to depend on the targets' relative timing. The presence of a foveal stimulus overlapping in time with the onset of a peripheral target can be shown to have an inhibitory effect on saccades (Fischer 1986). Conversely, a temporal gap between the offset of a central stimulus and the onset of a peripheral target, can substantially shorten saccadic latencies (Saslow 1967). The disappearance of the fixation target during the gap is thought to produce an automatic disengagement of attention, thereby by-passing one of the processes that contribute to the latency (Fischer 1986; Posner and Petersen 1990). This disengagement is believed to depend on extrastriate mechanisms. This means that we would expect latencies in the 'overlap' condition to become shorter

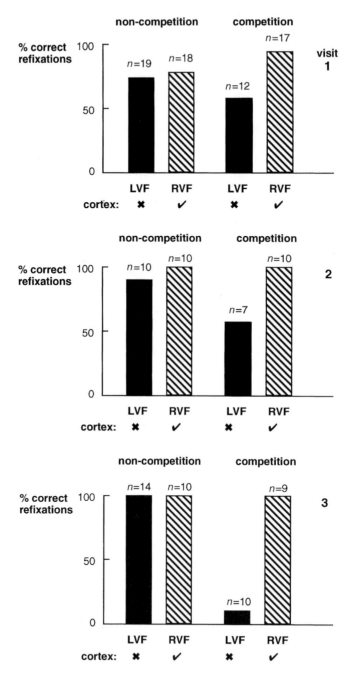

Fig. 8.3 Fixation shift results for child (PP) who has undergone early hemispherectomy to relieve intractable epilepsy. In this figure 50% correct response is at chance. His behaviour was above chance for targets on both the left and the right on non-competition, but only above chance on the right side of space in competition.

with age as cortical disengagement mechanisms develop. Studies carried out by Bruce Hood (1991; Hood and Atkinson 1993) on infants over the first six post-term months, using these gap paradigms, support this prediction. Saccadic latencies generally reduced with age, but this reduction was significantly greater in 'overlap' than in 'gap' conditions.

In adults, attentional shifts can be affected if stimuli are presented in rapid sequences. For example, a prior target to which subjects briefly switch attention, even without an overt orienting response, can either facilitate or inhibit a subsequent response to the same location, depending on the time interval (Posner 1980). The inhibitory effect (called 'inhibition of return' or IOR), in particular, has been argued to depend heavily on collicular mechanisms, on the basis of reported nasal–temporal asymmetries (Rafal *et al*. 1989, 1991) and on data showing that there is interference with IOR from collicular damage in progressive supranuclear palsy (Posner *et al*. 1985). Unlike adults, infants cannot be told that they should not orient to the first target; but the competition effect can be exploited to prevent them doing so to a brief target. This paradigm has provided evidence for both facilitation and inhibition of return, at different temporal intervals in 6 month olds and in adults, but these two effects have not been found in 3 month olds (Hood 1993; Hood and Atkinson 1991). Johnson and Tucker (1993), using slightly different stimuli, found IOR in 4 month olds but not in 2 month olds. These results suggest the interactions leading to IOR and facilitation do not arise from the same cortical modules controlling visual behaviour which first become operational between birth and 3 months. An element of caution is required here. The facilitatory and inhibitory effects we have been discussing are not all-or-nothing effects, switched off and on depending on a particular time interval between onset and offset of stimuli. The effects are also dependent on the detailed stimulus characteristics and interactions between these characteristics of the different targets. An example of this is that in a recent report, IOR effects have been demonstrated in newborns when the appropriate stimulus conditions and temporal parameters have been used (Valenza *et al*. 1994). This result also rather worryingly casts doubt on our ideas of identifying the mechanisms of IOR with cortical areas, in that we have previously argued that such cortical loops are unlikely to be operational in the newborn period.

In conclusion, from all these studies of attentional shifts, we have suggested that, by analogy with adult modelling, the change in attentional control between 1 and 3 months is likely to be related to the onset of function at about 3 months of age of attentional mechanisms involving superior colliculus, striate, and extrastriate connections (as shown in Fig. 8.1). The newborn's behaviour is usually under subcortical control (Atkinson and Braddick 1985; Braddick and Atkinson 1988), although there may be certain limited conditions where cortical functioning can be demonstrated. The inability of newborns to shift fixation to a peripheral target, if a central target is already fixated, is very similar to what is called 'sticky fixation' in a neurological condition of 'Balint's syndrome'. The patient does not suffer from 'neglect' or optic apraxia but rather lacks the co-ordination of mechanisms controlling saccadic eye movements and selective attention, to provide accurate spatial localizing. Balint's syndrome involves bilateral lesions in parieto-occipital areas, but may also involve the circuitry between the superior colliculus and parietal lobes for controlling shifts of attention (review by de Renzi 1982). Very similar behaviour to Balint's patients has been seen in primates with bilateral parietal damage (Mountcastle 1978). Schiller (1985) has also reported similar deficits with damage to the superior colliculus and frontal eye fields. Again, the evidence for the development of cortical streams lends support to the idea that crude localizing of single targets can be carried out by subcortical collicular mechanisms, while more elaborate selective processes, to shift attention from one object to another, require executive control from the striate and extrastriate cortex. These latter networks are also likely to involve the pulvinar, for linking subcortical and cortical areas. Recent theoretical considerations of the feedback and feedforward loops between cortical and thalamic areas, including the pulvinar (Crick and Koch 1998), do suggest that with the discovery of multiple subdivisions of the subcortical areas and multiple feedback loops to the cortex, the simple account offered here for attentional development may turn out to be only a small part of the complete story.

8.4.1.2 *Changes in the pattern of scanning eye movements with age*

Inferences about development of attention have been made from monitoring changes in eye scanning patterns, varying age, and the type of stimulus used. A number of studies have looked at changes in spontaneous eye scanning patterns with age (Maurer and Salapatek 1976; Bronson 1990; Hainline 1993). Bronson suggested that newborns in the first 6 weeks of life make many unguided scanning movements interspersed with long periods when a single target is fixated. Older infants scan between the features of targets in static displays and make more accurate target-elicited saccades than newborns. Bronson also claimed that if the target is dynamic then the amount of scanning between features is reduced; the infant tends to fixate a single flickering target for relatively long periods of time in a way similar to the scanning patterns of newborns. From these results, Bronson proposed that a phylogenetically older subcortical system was operating for dynamic stimuli and a cortical mechanism, which can inhibit eye movement control of the older system, is required to allow targets to be selected for attention. Hainline (1993), however, found no consistent changes in scanning patterns either in type or latency in the first 3 months of life and suggested that many of the earlier findings were related to posture and state of arousal which is clearly easier to control, and is stable for longer periods of time, in older infants compared with newborns (see discussion in Chapter 2). Her argument is that if newborns were in a rather more drowsy state for much of the time compared with 3 month olds, then they might show reduced eye scanning patterns in spontaneous looking.

As yet there are very few data collected longitudinally to measure changes in spontaneous fixation durations and eye scanning patterns with age. What is more, the variation across infants can often mask, in cross-sectional studies, the possible general changes in fixation patterns which may take place, as the infant grows older. However in one study, where visual attention was measured in infants, followed longitudinally from birth through to 6 months of age, it was found that fixation durations initially rose from levels measured in the newborn, to peak at 2 months, before reducing again (Hood *et al.* 1994). This might suggest that the eye movement control mechanisms, reflecting attention, may be different or differentially functional at different ages during the first 6 months of life.

A number of early studies have claimed that spontaneous eye scanning patterns in newborns and 1 month olds are concentrated around the external contour of a pattern, whereas older infants scan both external and internal contours (Maurer and Salapatek 1976; Haith *et al.* 1977). Haith *et al.* suggested that this 'capturing' of attention by the outer contours is a built-in mechanism to provide maximum neural firing (the outer contour being of higher overall contrast than the inner contours by virtue of its extensive high contrast edges).

The external contour of a pattern is also claimed to have a special role in the attention of newborn infants in explaining the so-called 'externality' effect (Milewski 1976). In habituation studies, if the new pattern has an identical outer contour to the old pattern (to which the infant is habituated) then the newborn may fail to discriminate between the old and the new patterns (this has already been discussed under 'face perception' in Chapter 4 on newborns). The circumstances under which this effect is manifest are thought to tell us about the relative attentional salience of the outer and inner contours of the pattern, i.e. the features of the pattern to which the infant has selectively attended in the process of habituation. Ian Bushnell, in our group, many years ago found that the externality effect could be nullified if the inner contours were made dynamic while the outer ones stayed stationary (Bushnell 1979). This is reminiscent of Bronson's findings on the persistent fixation of dynamic targets. Haith's theory of neural firing could also be applied to the finding that when the inner contour is dynamic (i.e. flickering or moving) and the outer contour stationary, then the externality effect is negated, because of the relatively higher overall rate of neuronal firing produced by a dynamic stimulus rather than a stationary one. The dynamic stimulus thus 'wins' in capturing the infant's attention.

Of course the externality effect, whereby the outer contour captures the infant's attention and causes the child to have reduced sensitivity to internal contours of patterns, may not necessarily be an effect which disappears by the end of infancy. An effect, possibly related to the externality effect is called *lateral masking* or *visual crowding*, which has been studied in pre-school children rather than infants (Atkinson *et al.* 1986*a*, 1987, 1988*a*; Anker *et al.* 1989; Atkinson 1991, 1993), and this has been developed as a clinical test called the Cambridge Crowding Cards (described in Chapter 2). In a typical 'crowded' display a single letter has a ring of different letters surrounding it laterally and the child is asked to select and attend to the letter in the centre of the display and ignore the letters surrounding it. Usually, the child is asked either to name the centre letter or to match it visually to one of a number of possible letters. There is a change with age in the ability of children to ignore the irrelevant surrounding letters and select the central one for visual matching. To measure the extent of crowding, a comparison is made between the size needed for accurate visual matching of an isolated letter, compared with the minimum size of letter, when surrounded by other letters or patterns. This ratio is called the *crowding ratio*, and varies with the stimulus parameters of both the central letter and its surround.

For letter displays, the small crowding effect normally seen in adults is also shown by most 6 year olds; younger children show much larger crowding effects. Interestingly, some dyslexics also show marked crowding effects under certain stimulus conditions (Atkinson 1991, 1993). In many clinical conditions, such as in children with Williams' syndrome, their crowding ratios look like those of normal 4 year olds, although their chronological age is well above 4 years. This result does not reflect that they have a mental age of 4 years, as many of the Williams' syndrome children have much higher verbal mental age equivalents, close to their chronological age. Such effects can be thought of as selective attentional problems rather than a simple loss of visual contrast sensitivity or acuity. Selective attention must also be important in tests of embedded figures (such as those mentioned in Chapter 2 in the Atkinson Battery of Child Development for Examining Functional Vision or ABCDEFV tests). However, a united theoretical account of the processing involved in producing crowding effects across these different tests has not been put forward in any detail.

In conclusion, we see that the data from spontaneous eye scanning eye movements on infants is at present rather limited and at times controversial. One problem with all studies using eye scanning patterns to consider attentional processing is that as yet, there is very little consensus as to what the exact relationship between spontaneous eye movements and adult attention is or means in terms of selective mechanisms. However, recent studies of the eye movements made by adults in conjunction with a goal-directed motor act (e.g. by Mike Land and Mary Hayhoe and their colleagues (Land and Hayhoe, 1999)where the spontaneous eye movements and fixations made while making a peanut butter and jelly sandwich have been analysed) may be a more revealing paradigm to lead us to a more direct theory to link attentional eye movements to behaviour. Models derived in this way may, in the future, be useful in making sense of any changes in the nature of spontaneous scanning eye movement patterns made by infants at different ages.

8.4.1.3 *Measures of changes in focusing accuracy or accommodation to targets attended*

In general when adults attend to an object they not only foveate it, they also adjust their accommodation (using the ciliary muscles to alter the curvature and hence focusing power of the lens) to bring the image into sharp focus. Development of accommodation has already been discussed in Chapter 5. Some newborn infants do shift their focus in the appropriate direction in depth for a target moved towards them or away from them, but they do not do this with great accuracy or very reliably, and the range over which they change their focus is limited to near space (about 75 cm away from their eyes). Only approximately 50% of newborns consistently accommodated in and out to 75 cm, when tested on three to five separate occasions in a 5-min testing period (Braddick *et al.* 1979). By 3 months of age, nearly all infants accommodate consistently over near distances, and by 6 months of age infants accommodate out to about at least 150 cm. By analogy to measures of the lateral visual field mentioned above, the idea of an effective visual attentional field can be considered, measured on the midline in terms of target distance for initiating changes of accommodation. It seems that this attentional field also increases with age and may be subject to the same constraints as those affecting the extent of the lateral visual field.

In a number of studies of children with neurological deficits it was found that children show poor shifts of accommodation for targets at different distances (e.g. Atkinson 1989). Often these children also show inability to make saccadic shifts to peripherally located targets in the fixation shift paradigm and show reduced lateral visual fields, particularly in competition conditions when both a foveal and peripheral target are presented together. In a large cohort study of over 100 children identified at the Hammersmith Hospital in the first weeks of life with indicators of potential perinatal brain damage (Mercuri *et al.* 1995, 1997*a,b*), it was found that for those with extensive brain damage (hypoxic–ischaemic encephalopathy grades 2 or 3) there was a strong likelihood of poor accommodative responses and deficits on the fixation shift paradigm, whereas for children with early focal lesions there is a much lower probability of these early indicators of attentional deficits. Nevertheless, it seems extremely likely that for infants in either of these groups, these early indicators of deficits or delay will be correlated with at least milder forms of attentional deficit at a later stage.

Using measurements of accommodation to gauge attentional shifts is a relatively new idea, and it is not known, as yet, how well it correlates with other measures of attention, particularly for older children and adults. In a second infant vision screening programme in Cambridge (described more fully in Chapter 5) measures of accommodation were used to indicate likely hyperopic refractive errors. The idea is that these infants show poor accommodation because the accommodative effort, required to gain a sharp image, is very great due to their large hyperopic refractive errors (i.e. the resting state of the eye is very long-sighted). Other infants, identified at screening because of their poor accommodation, do not show marked degrees of long-sightedness when refracted under cycloplegia. It may be that this lack of appropriate accommodation in the latter group is an indicator of poorer attentional control than their peers. It remains to be seen how this group of poor accommodators develop and whether these early indicators are predictive of other attentional losses at school age, such as ADHD. These infants are the subject of an intensive longitudinal follow-up study which should start to yield outcome results in the next year or two.

8.4.2 Overall conclusions on early attentional eye and head movement systems

In conclusion, a consistent picture of attentional development is emerging from these three rather different measures of eye movement control. In normal development, the subcortically controlled newborn system is gradually, but rapidly, replaced by a number of cortical to subcortical controlling circuits in the first 6 months of life. Each circuit, controlling accommodation, shifts of fixation, and sustained attention, must be interlinked to others, as well as develop within themselves. Inhibitory as well as excitatory links must be developed. These processes start in the first few postnatal months, but take many years to fully mature to adult levels.

8.5 DEVELOPMENT OF VISUALLY GUIDED REACHING AND GRASPING

The second attention and action system to be developed, which needs to be linked to the head and eye movement systems considered above, is that controlling reaching and grasping in young infants. In this section the development of reaching and grasping is discussed, starting with a brief overview of some controversial issues and going on to our own research in this area. The motor aspects of these abilities have started to be intensely studied in recent years. The linking of these motor abilities to more cognitive aspects of development has also been well represented in the work of Piaget, particularly with respect to object permanence tasks. However, the detailed understanding of how the infants analyse objects in terms of visual attributes and attentional salience, and then integrate this analysis with motor acts, is much less well explored.

8.5.1 Controversies in development of reaching and grasping

There has been some controversy in the past 20 years over neonatal reaching and grasping. The results from several early studies by Tom Bower and his colleagues (Bower *et al.* 1970; Bower 1972) suggested that neonates adjusted their reaches in an attempt to touch solid objects, in terms of both direction of reach and in the aperture of the fingers (hand shaping) as the arm approached the object. In addition, Bower claimed that newborns reached more to objects within arm's reach than to objects out of reach and more to solid real objects than to photographs of the same objects. However, researchers carrying out later studies failed to replicate many of these findings in newborns and pointed out methodological problems in many of the early Bower studies (e.g. DiFranco *et al.* 1978; Ruff and Halton 1978; Rader and Stern 1982). A number of Bower's claims have been supported by other researchers, but for infants over 3 months of age (e.g. Bruner and Klossowski, 1972, on coarse hand shaping).

Trevarthen (1974) claimed, like Bower, that infants made pre-reaching movements towards objects, but he considered these movements as pre-functional rather than truly functional. His ideas were an early form of the 'two visual systems' theory, with suggestions of pre-functional, subcortical orienting in newborns followed by functional cortical activity in later reaching. Pre-reaching was considered, along with eye movements, as a component of a single orienting response. One of the most detailed studies of neonatal responses to visual stimuli was carried out by Claus von Hofsten (1982). He found that many of the arm movements made by infants while fixating objects were towards the object. This was not the case if the infant was not fixating the object. This does suggest visually guided pre-reaching movements present shortly after birth, but he did not find any of the sophisticated responses found by Bower in newborns (e.g. hand shaping). In general, his results were in agreement with Colwyn Trevarthen's; neonatal pre-reaching was part of a general orienting response and this orienting could be driven by either vision or touch.

Intentional reaching is generally thought to emerge from 3 to 4 months onwards in normal infants (von Hofsten 1984). Several measures have been taken as indicators of this changeover from pre-reaching to true reaching. At the transition point between pre-reaching and reaching there have been reports of fidgety movements (Haddersalgra and Prechtl 1992) and this has been seen by some to represent the breakdown of orienting responses, which are replaced by the infant's attempts to execute a number of different cortically controlled actions in a sequence.

One aspect of this breakdown is the uncoupling of synergistic movements of the arm and hand found in pre-reaching. Individual components of the reach and grasp become manifest with the reach usually consisting of at least two segments in terms of velocity peaks—a first reaching peak followed by the grasping stage. In many instances the reaching component itself is divided into a number of segments, each with their own velocity peak, the number of segments depending on the salience of the object, its distance and its position relative to the starting position of the hand (von Hofsten 1979, 1991; Mounoud and Vintner 1981).

There has been considerable debate concerning the extent to which infants look at the hand and target during a reach. Some have claimed a constant switching of fixation from hand to object (e.g. White *et al.* 1964). However, others, such as Trevarthen (1974) and von Hofsten (1991) have found that very early pre-reaching is ballistic, involving only essentially one movement. This may be due to the newborn's limited capacity to switch attention to and fro from hand to object. It is thought that by 4 months of age reaching is under visual guidance, in that infants can use visual feedback to modify their reach (Mc Donnell 1975; Bower 1976). The detailed longitudinal study by von Hofsten (1979) went some way in resolving these issues. He found that at about 6 months of age the largely zig-zagging approach to objects had disappeared, the number of segments in the reach dropped steadily up to 9 months, but the relative length of each segment changed with age. In early reaching the zigzagging segments were all of approximately the same duration, whereas with later reaching the first segment had increased to about 500 ms followed by a series of short segments (about 250 ms). The first segment covered an increasing percentage of the approach with age, up to about 75% of the reach by 9 months of age. This has been seen by Jeannerod (1988) as a gradual separation of the reach into two segments, an initial transport segment (possibly becoming smooth and ballistic with practice) followed by smaller correcting movements for grasping as the hand nears the target. However, an unresolved issue is the extent of visual control in very early reaching— von Hofsten did not find extensive looking between the hand and object as had earlier been claimed and has argued that other sources of information, such as proprioception and kinaesthesis, define the position of the hand. Only beyond 6 months was visual feedback used to correct the reach.

The other area of controversy is on the age of onset of hand shaping in grasping. Bower (1972) and Trevarthen (1974) argue for changes of hand aperture appropriate to size in newborns, while von Hofsten and Ronquist (1988), among others, argue for much later onsets (at the earliest in some infants at 9 months of age). George Butterworth and his colleagues (1997) have recently presented infants with different size objects on strings and measured the number of whole hand grips at different ages. The number of whole hand grips diminished with age showing that precision grips develop later than power grips (as suggested by Halverson 1937) and infants used more fingers to grasp an object as the object increased in size. However, as the infants tended to grasp all the objects presented to them, Butterworth *et al.* were unable to find any variability in likelihood of reaching which was dependent on object size.

There is also relatively late development of hand adjustment in orientation in anticipation of the grip on different shaped objects (Lockman *et al.* 1984; von Hofsten and Fazel-Dandy 1984). For many everyday tasks, adult-like adjustment of the arm and hand approach for lifting an object is not seen reliably until 6–8 years of age (Smyth and Mason 1997) and other aspects of grasping and lifting (grasp/power grip ratio) have also been found to be relatively late in maturing (Forssberg *et al.* 1991).

8.6 SUBCORTICAL AND CORTICAL MOTOR PATHWAYS

As already said, it is difficult in development to separate visual, attentional, and motor limitations. Nevertheless, it is important to know about the motor system in early life so that the extent of motor limitations can be gauged. From the extensive studies of Kuypers and his colleagues on non-human primates (Kuypers 1962; Lawrence and Kuypers 1968), we believe that the ventromedial subcortical system is involved primarily in integration of movements of the limbs and trunk, the lateral subcortical system is involved in independent hand movements and the ability to flex the thumb, and the cortical pyramidal system controls distal movements of the hand and independent finger movements. Studies on adults with lesions of the cerebral cortex support the notion of separate circuits for the distal and proximal parts of the reach (Jeannerod 1986).

In human development, there is an initial coupling of flexion of the arm and fisting of the hand. This synergy is relaxed at about 2–4 months. In infants the pincer grasp (present usually at about 1 year of age) has been taken as a marker of corticomotor neuronal functioning. Recently, data from transcranial magnetic stimulation has provided a direct non-invasive measure of corticospinal development and suggests a relatively low level of activity initially in corticomotor neurons in newborns, followed by marked improvements towards the end of the first year of life (Eyre *et al.* 1991; Watts *et al.* 1992).

Recently, there have been extensive anatomical and electrophysiological studies on primate cortical systems for reaching and grasping (excellently reviewed by Milner and Goodale 1995; Jeannerod 1988; Rizzolatti *et al.* 1997). The circuits to be discussed are schematized in Fig. 8.4.

Four main areas are of prime importance: the posterior parietal complex around the intraparietal sulcus; the prefrontal and frontal areas; the premotor and motor cortex; circuits involving the cerebellum and subcortical areas. In particular, the intraparietal and ventral parietal areas (AIP and VIP), and frontal areas F5 and F4 (in Brodman area 6) are important in reaching and grasping. AIP contains both visual-dominant and motor-dominant neurons (e.g. see Sakata *et al.* 1992) and is an area where neurons are primarily sensitive to object properties and specific actions

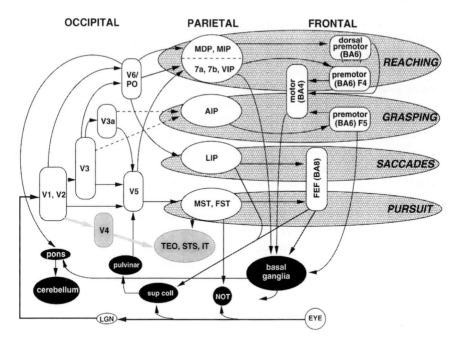

Fig. 8. 4 The neural circuitry, thought to be involved in different action systems. This figure is based on data from primate studies and case history studies of adults with specific brain damage.

towards them. It projects forward to F5. Jeannerod (1988) suggests that this network is particularly important in grasping. Rizzolatti *et al.* (1997) suggest that AIP provides multiple descriptions of an object and the actions towards it and that F5 selects the most appropriate action (for example, depending on the purpose of the action and position of other objects). VIP also contains visual- and action-specific neurons (Colby *et al.* 1993, Bremmer *et al.* 1997) which are strongly dependent on the direction and speed of the object's movement. Many of them show spatial constancy, i.e. they generalize over gaze direction. VIP projects to F4 and seems likely to be involved in reaching. Rizzolatti and his co-researchers have emphasized populations of neurons whose firing is correlated with particular goal-related motor acts, some are related to reaching and some to grasping. The prefrontal neurons are not retinally tuned but are defined in terms of body coordinates and so are independent of eye position.

Gentilucci and Rizzolatti (1990) have considered various co-ordinate systems which could be used to describe active movements. It seems that movements are planned as a series of straight trajectories which are then translated into complex movements between the joints. A number of studies of the kinetics of development of reaching have made the segmental nature of the reach clearer, with changes of curvature being found at the transitions between segments (e.g. Matthew and Cook 1990; von Hofsten 1991; Thelen *et al.* 1993; Konczak and Thelen 1994). In general, the variability of intralimb positioning and organization of grasping reduces with age. This variability may go some way to explain the differences in description of early reaching from different studies. By 2 years, many spatial and temporal end-point and proximal joint parameters exhibit a variability close to or within the adult range, although immaturities may remain well into childhood depending on the difficulties of the movements (Konczak and Dichgans 1997).

By about 7 months of age normal infants start to be able to sit unsupported by an adult. There have been a number of studies investigating the relationship between the developmental changes in reaching and independent sitting. For example, Rochat (1992) found that infants in a stage before independent sitting tended to have synergistically coupled bimanual reaches whereas unilateral reaching developed alongside independent sitting. Presumably, bimanual reaching is more likely to be successful than unilateral, if your base position (of the back and bottom) tends to be unstable. However, it is difficult to know from these correlations whether the trunk control determines the hand movements, as part of a learning process, or whether the two (bimanual hand synergy and trunk control) are initially controlled by one mechanism with the maturation of a mechanism for unilateral hand control being paralleled by, but not causally related to, a mechanism controlling multiple stable rotations around the trunk to enable independent sitting. It is clear, however, that with better trunk control the infant is able to extend exploration of space with the hands, which in turn presumably acts as a trigger to more sophisticated body movements for crawling.

8.6.1 Reaching under binocular and monocular viewing

We have started to look at what visual cues are used to guide reaching in infancy. In particular, we have looked at whether disparity cues are used to guide reaching, by measuring the course of visually guided reaches in infants who have just started reaching (6–9 month olds) and comparing their ability with both eyes viewing, to a situation where one eye is covered (Braddick *et al.* 1996a). If stereoscopic information is used to control reaching, then covering one eye should reduce the accuracy or efficiency of the reach. This was the first study to use the Elite motion analysing system in human infants. The system involves video tracking of lightweight reflectors on the skin to register and analyse the three-dimensional trajectory, velocity, and timing of a limb movement. Its advantage over other systems is that there are no trailing wires and very lightweight reflectors. Its disadvantage is that there is a risk of infants finding the lightweight reflectors more interesting than the targets, even to the extent of attempting to eat the reflectors!

At 6–9 months of age, a reaching action frequently consists of a number of segments, each segment defined by an acceleration followed by a deceleration. The most extreme case of this is where the hand comes almost to rest in an incorrect position, and this mis-reach is then followed by one or more corrective movements. Thus an increased number of segments indicates greater inaccuracy and uncertainty in the initial ballistic action. Our results show a tendency for an increased number of segments, and also higher peak velocity, to occur in monocular viewing conditions compared with binocular viewing (see Fig. 8.5). These results imply that binocular information contributes to the infant's representation of three-dimensional space and is used to guide rapid and appropriate actions.

It should be noted that these differences in reaching between monocular and binocular viewing for infants are not quite the same as the difference which has been reported between monocular and binocular viewing conditions in adults (Servos *et al.* 1992). The visual control of reaching in infants at this age is still immature in many respects compared with the adult.

8.6.2 Preferential looking and preferential reaching in early development

Over the past 5 years a number of studies have been carried out in our laboratory on early reaching and grasping in young normal infants (e.g. King *et al.* 1996), to start to look at the interaction between the attentional salience of particular objects and the likelihood of the infant reaching to them. This has been largely the work of John King and Chris Newman in our group.

To reach out for an object involves encoding its location. Here the parameters are the direction and amplitude of the arm movement. To grasp an object, on the other hand, requires coding of intrinsic features of an object such as its size, shape, and orientation (Arbib 1985; Jeannerod 1988). In addition, to grasp successfully, the two elements must be temporally coupled. Now it is quite possible that, as we have suggested above, the two systems of reaching and grasping may use different circuitry, and these two may not be well coupled in the early development of reaching and grasping. In addition, there is the attentional system for orienting the head and eyes for objects in space and the cortical system for switching visual attention from one object to another (discussed above). This means that when we present the young infant with an object which can be reached for, we have potentially five systems operating: one subcortical system for orienting to sudden change in stimulation; a largely

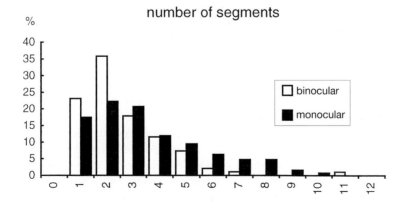

Fig. 8.5 Comparison of the number of segments in monocular and binocular reaches.

ventral stream system for discriminating one object from another (including possibly size discrimination); a dorsal action system operating for switching the head and eyes from one object to another; a dorsal action system controlling reaching; and a dorsal action system for controlling grasping. In primate studies the neurological underpinnings of these systems contain overlapping but distinct components. However, in human adults these systems are synchronized and operate in unison, with different systems taking priority to control actions, depending on the particular goals of our actions. In Chapters 3 and 6, and in this chapter, the development of these different ventral and dorsal systems has been discussed as though they were all completely separate in development. A good argument has been put forward for mechanisms controlling orienting to operate at birth, with ventral stream mechanisms for size and orientation coming into action relatively early, and striate and extrastriate mechanisms, which form the basis of motion discrimination and depth perception (dorsal stream), a little later. Earlier in this chapter there were discussions on what is known about early development of reaching and hand shaping in grasping, and what changes in ability in reaching and grasping come in towards the end of the first year of life.

However, very little detailed study has been made of how these systems interact with one another during development and whether any system takes priority in controlling attention and action. A recent set of studies in our unit has looked at the development of these five systems to control reaching and looking preferences in infants from the beginning of reaching at 5 months through to 15 months of age. In these studies one system's priorities are pitched against another, to see if these priorities change during development so that one system comes to 'decide' the final actions carried out by the infant.

The paradigm used has been relatively simple. Pairs of small red solid lightweight plastic cylinders have been placed at arm's length from the infant and preferential looking (which cylinder they look at first) and preferential reaching (which cylinder they first touch and attempt to grasp) have been recorded. The cylinders vary in size (small—1 cm diameter, medium—2.5 cm diameter and large—6 cm diameter). For nearly all infants below 10 months of age the large cylinder is ungraspable with one hand alone, because of their small hand size.

8.6.3 Preferential reaching

In one previous published study there has been the suggestion that the size of object affected the *likelihood* of reaching for it (Siddiqui 1995), although in this study very few reaches were elicited at all from 5 to 9 month olds. In our study we give the infant a choice of two objects to reach for, thus avoiding trials where there was no reaching or looking. In addition to their choice, we have recorded many aspects of the kinematics of reaching and grasping using the Elite infrared monitoring system. Results to date suggest several very interesting transitions in both attention and motor systems in the first year of life, implying that there are different priorities in attentional action systems which decide behaviour at different stages during development. In several studies there was a significant preference for reaching to the smaller diameter cylinder of the pair between 6 and 12 months of life (King *et al.* 1996, 1998). This can be seen in Fig. 8.6.

It is not always seen in very early reaches of infants and is not seen in older infants about 1 year (by which time all three cylinder sizes are small enough to allow many infants to hold the object in one hand). It would appear that there is developing ability to use visual information to predict the 'graspability' of objects. Infants between 8 and 11 months also appear to look longer at objects before they reach, than either younger or older infants. When one looks at the kinematics of reaching in this middle age group, they also seem to show a slower peak velocity and movement duration with a longer acceleration time and an increased number of velocity peaks. These changes starting at about 7–8 months suggest that infants may be starting to use more elaborate planning strategies, gained from information concerning the detailed visual aspects of objects, as they grow older, and that once these circuits have started to become active they can once again speed up in their reaching and grasping at about 1 year of age, becoming accomplished unimanual reachers by this age. In addition, by 1 year of age they can sit unaided and make rotational movements of the trunk and these new capacities make unimanual reaching easier than at previous ages.

8.6.4 Preferential looking

In an early study, using 2D simulations of the 3D cylinders on computer screens, it was found that infants tended to look at the larger diameter cylinder first (King

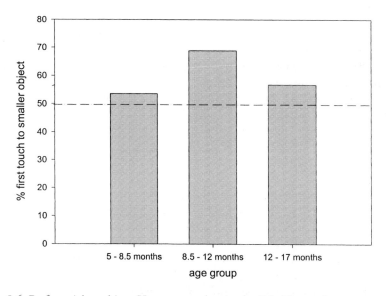

Fig. 8.6 Preferential reaching. Here we see that in the 8.5–12 month age group there is a clear reaching preference for the smaller (graspable) cylinder. Note that 50% is the chance level. The preference is not significantly different from chance in children over 1 year, whose hands are large enough to grasp the large cylinder, nor in the youngest age group.

1998). However, this result was dependent on the exact distance of the edge of the cylinders from a fixation spot in the centre of the computer screen and the larger diameter cylinder was clearly nearer to the initial fixation point than the smaller diameter cylinders. We decided that this could be taken as evidence of the subcortical visual orienting system (largely collicular responses) making a differential response to the nearer of two objects in the lateral field. Indeed, it is generally believed that young infants will orient to the nearer of two peripheral stimuli in classic clinical orthoptic perimetry testing in the test of *confrontation,* for measuring the extent of lateral fields (when simultaneously a target is brought inwards on both the left and right to centre). Of course there are important differences between real 3D objects and the 2D renderings on computer screens used in our experiments and it is possible that infants detected that the stimuli were not truly 3D and that this affected their preferential looking behaviour. However, when 3D real solid cylinders were used in later experiments, rather than the 2D renderings, it was found that very young infants (5–8 months) once again tended to look first at the large cylinder rather than the medium or small cylinder, with which it was paired, and that they were more likely to reach for it, if they first looked at it (Fig. 8.7).

Thus there seems to be a synergy between the looking and reaching attentional systems initially, and possibly use of the same output system. Hofsten (1991) and Gauthier *et al.* (1998) have both commented on this type of coupling in the neonate and, of course, this system may still be operating at this later age in early reaching. This linked synergy between preferential looking and preferential reaching gradually

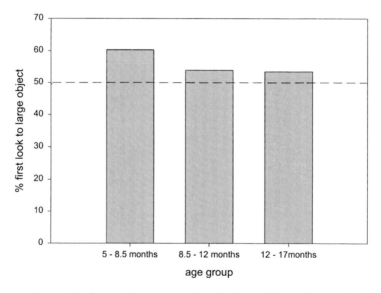

Fig. 8.7 Preferential looking. When presented with a large (6.5 cm diameter) and a small (1 cm diameter) cylinder, infants of 5–8.5 months tended to look at the *larger* diameter cylinder first.

breaks down with age, so that the properties pertaining to the size of the hand relative to the object diameter ('graspability') start to be those involved in controlling the action system. At this stage in development the two mechanisms are splitting off from each other— what the infant might like to look at first is not necessarily the same as the object of preference in reaching. It is as though the goal of the grasping action becomes more important and salient than the goal of the preferential looking system, although both may still be operating at the same moment in the infant's brain. It is perhaps another example of the higher-level extrastriate cortical systems taking over from lower level orienting systems.

8.6.5 Right/left looking biases

There is another curious preference which we have found in these infant reaching experiments. In many of our studies a transient right spatial bias in first looks has been found, which is superimposed on the other preferences. (An example is shown in Fig. 8.8). Whether this represents a significant superiority of the orienting mechanism for the right side of space, indicating a mechanism which is more active in the left hemisphere rather than right at an early age, is not known. A relation to mechanisms leading to eventual right-handedness is another possibility. There are a number of right biases already noted in the literature in earlier reflex behaviour, such as in the tonic neck reflex (Bishop 1990).

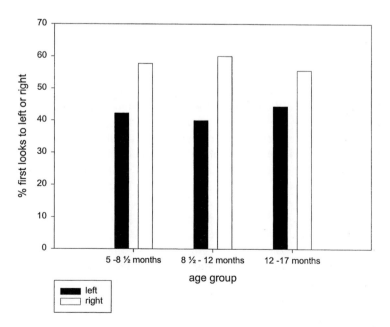

Fig. 8. 8 There is a bias in looking at the object on the right of fixation shift, no matter what the size of the cylinder.

8.6.6 Ipsilateral reaching to the object on the same side as the reaching hand

A marked bias towards reaches that do not cross the infant's body midline (ipsilateral reaching) is seen throughout the data collected on reaching in the first year of life. Bruner (1969) was one of the first to comment on this 'midline barrier'. However, most infants over 5 months of age can successfully reach across the midline for a single object in line with the side of their body contralateral to the reaching hand (Provine and Westerman 1979), but they do not choose to do this if there is another object on the ipsilateral side in line with the reaching hand. Dorothy Bishop (1990) notes that split-brain adult patients show the same ipsilateral bias, and we have seen this bias in a number of infants with unilateral brain damage and in acallosal patients. Bishop's argument is that development of the callosal crossings allows inhibition of this ipsilateral bias. Contralateral reaching involves an extra 'cost' in time for inhibitory processes, and requires better biomechanical control of the arm and rotation of the trunk, than that necessary for ipsilateral reaching. As young infants who have just started reaching will have limitations in all these systems, it is not surprising to see the ipsilateral bias, but impossible to know which type of immaturity is most limiting and is causing the bias. As we saw this bias even in infants up to 18 months of age, it is tempting to consider the callosal immaturities to be the most important rather than control of trunk rotation. However, as it is faster (shorter duration) and easier biomechanically even for adults to reach ipsilaterally, such factors cannot be ignored as limitations in the developing infant, and must also form some restraint on contralateral reaches. The most 'natural' reaching may always be bimanual in young infants and it is of course possible that we have merely observed half of a bimanual reach in limiting the infants' reaching in these studies to the use of one hand.

In summary, the preferential reaching measures provide us with a model of the infant's changing priorities in terms of the output of the five attention and action systems I discussed earlier in the chapter. We can speculate that systems, analogous to those found in the parietal–frontal circuits of primates for gauging 'graspability' and programming reaches, first start to operate at about 7–9 months of age. Before this time infants younger than 8 months seem to show a preferential looking bias towards the large object (6 cm diameter cylinder), and this looking pattern must be suppressed so that the infant is linking their looking and reaching to the same 'graspable' object. There may also be the massive ipsilateral side bias to overcome in preferring to reach for an object which is graspable and liftable, and while this ipsilateral side bias persists in unimanual reaches up to 18 months of age, if the child's hand is large enough to grasp even the 6 cm diameter cylinder, then there will be no preference for any particular size and merely a preponderance of ipsilateral reaches. As ipsilateral compared with contralateral reaches are always easier even in adulthood, it would seem that we can speculate that the mechanisms of dominant right hand reaching and grasping must end up with stronger, more reliable operational circuits at some stage of development. From previous studies, the age of dominant right hand use for reaching and grasping will depend to some extent on the goal of the reach (Bishop 1990). For an object which is easy to reach and grasp (in nearby space and of graspable size with a non-slippery surface) children up to 4–5 years often use either hand. More detailed studies of the period between 2 and 5 years are needed to measure the dependence of hand use on object properties. In general, the infant is continuously improving a flexible planning action system from the time of early reaches to adult maturity. The attentional salience system, initially dominated by mechanisms within the object recognition stream, needs to be adjusted to take into account the affordances of objects related to their graspability properties. It makes ecological sense for the young child to learn about and use the visual properties of objects which are more likely to be graspable. It may not be an accident that the sweets called 'Smarties' or 'M and Ms' are popular particularly with toddlers who have a good ventral stream object recognition system and have developed an accurate pincer grasp.

8.7 CONCLUSIONS

In the non-human primate visual system four different action/attention modules have been defined, each subserving a different aspect of behaviour. Earlier in this chapter, what is known about the areas involved in each of these modules was schematized in Fig. 8.4. What is known about the development of attention linked to two action streams has also been discussed—one for visuomotor selective attention (using head and eye movements), and one using arm and hand movements in addition to head and eye movements.

In development the system for saccadic tracking is already operational at birth, although this system is not totally reliable or accurate and only operates at slow velocities. This suggests that the underlying subcortical mechanisms are already wired up. These circuits are likely to involve the superior colliculus, basal ganglia, pulvinar, and cerebellum. These same subcortical mechanisms are operational for crude refixations in orienting to a peripheral target. Part of the evidence that they are subcortical comes from our studies on infants who have undergone hemispherectomy early in life and yet still orient to single peripheral stimuli to the side of space for which there are only subcortical control mechanisms (Braddick *et al.* 1992).

At about 3 months of age there are dramatic changes in the ability of infants to make rapid shifts of attention, using the saccadic foveation system in shifting atten-tion from one object of interest to another in an environment containing multiple objects. The underpinnings of this behaviour are highly likely to involve some parts of the parietal and frontal circuits shown in Fig. 8.2. Results from studies discussed in this chapter on *fixation shifts, fields,* and *inhibition of return* paradigms suggest that the parietal modules become active earlier than the frontal parts to which they are connected.

However, by 6 months of age the saccadic and pursuit modules, including their attentional inhibitory components, are functioning in an adult-like fashion, at least for displays in relatively nearby space to the infant. At this age some parts of the modules underpinning reaching and grasping start to be operational, but as these behaviours are highly immature until about 1 year to 18 months of age, it is clear that the motor and perceptual subsystems (including areas AIP, BA4, F4, and F6) develop relatively slowly over a period of years. The attentional foveating head and eye movement systems are not always well integrated with the attentional systems that are involved in reaching in these early stages. We have seen from our preferential reaching and preferential looking studies that there seems to be a period, about 6–9 months of age, when the attentional mechanisms, driving eye movements, may not be well synchronized with the attentional systems operating on affordances within the visuomotor arm and hand domain.

In turn, there are explanations purely in terms of immaturity of biomechanical subsystems (involving mechanisms controlling ipsilateral and contralateral reaching, and trunk stability) which have to be taken into account when considering early reaching and grasping. These proprioceptive and visual feedback mechanisms need in turn to be integrated with the attentional systems, to control mature, goal-directed reaching and grasping. Immaturity of parts of the frontal lobes may underpin behaviour where the infant fails to inhibit eye movements or hand movements to irrelevant distractors. However, even in adults, reaching trajectories to a target can be altered by distractor objects close to the target. It seems that this action system is always going to involve attentional selective and inhibitory mechanisms to calculate the most appropriate responses. This selection process will depend to some extent on attentional load (with load being greater the more distracting the non-targets are to the target). As yet it is very difficult to separate completely purely motor incompetence from limitations of selective attention and perhaps this is not a sensible division to make considering the number of potential feed-forward and feed-back circuits involved in these processes.

In Chapter 9 many ideas on normally developing action systems are linked to plasticity in development, when one of these systems has suffered a potential setback early in life. This can be due to abnormal genetic programming, peripheral factors affecting processing within the eye, or abnormal events early in life, such as lack of oxygen, affecting the visual brain. Often all four action systems (pursuit, saccadic shifts, reaching, and grasping) are found to be subtly affected, when the most sensitive measure is used for the particular stage of development which the child has reached. It makes no sense to try to separate out of these systems the attentional components. However, for identifying solutions in remediation for later problems in both the intellectual and visuomotor skills domains, it might be useful to identify the mechanisms (and neurological underpinnings) which were the starting point for setting off the cascade of abnormal development. This remediation may come from the understanding of abnormality in molecular and genetic terms, as well as our understanding at the systems level as described in this book.

9 Plasticity in visual development

In considering visual development there are a number of questions which arise perennially and are asked by both researchers and parents. One of the most important questions is how much variation is there in the course of visual development from one individual infant to another, and how is this variation brought about? An important practical question in this area is: how plastic are the brain connections underlying visual development? If some part of the visual brain cannot develop, because it either lacks the genetic programming or it has been damaged at an early stage, can other areas operate instead or can visual pathways develop later than normal in the recovery from damage? For example, can infants who have a very early-onset strabismus and abnormal binocular input ever develop normal three-dimensional vision? Does damage to specific brain areas other than those commonly thought of as in the classic visual pathway cause problems in visual development? Can early visual problems lead to permanent visuocognitive problems that affect the child's ability to read (i.e. can early visual problems lead to dyslexia)?

These questions have not as yet been very fully answered in the human case. However, there has been a substantial amount of very informative research with other species, providing analogous studies which add to the human clinical case studies in our attempt to answer these questions. From the primate work, we can guess at what the answers might be for some paediatric visual problems. What we cannot easily do at present is to decide how the particular peculiarities of being human might change this plasticity, either by limiting plasticity or expanding it in extent and time. From clinical work with abnormal paediatric populations we can see how visual development is changed, but we cannot yet have all the answers as to how to give successful treatment.

It would require an entire book to review systematically all the work with cats, primates, and other species on plasticity, and all the clinical studies on common paediatric visual problems such as cataract, congenital strabismus, and amblyopia. This chapter concentrates on our own work studying a number of different clinical populations in which vision has not developed along its normal course. Using these examples we are going to look at some of the current answers we can give to some of the questions on plasticity posed above. Plasticity will be considered under three broad headings:

1. Does extra or abnormal visual input produce changes in visual brain mechanisms?

2. Does abnormal input produce changes in development of more peripheral visual systems?

3. Does brain damage or abnormal brain structure produce compensating changes in other visual brain systems?

9.1 DOES EXTRA OR ABNORMAL VISUAL INPUT PRODUCE CHANGES IN VISUAL BRAIN DEVELOPMENT?

This is the perennial question in terms of sensitivity to environmental factors in the nature–nurture debate. Parents of children with normal vision, and of those with visual disability, always want to know whether the visual stimulation they give to their child will make any difference to the rate of visual development in eye–brain connections. In the case of human development it is easier to answer if abnormal visual input is discussed than if extra visual stimulation over and above that given in the normal environment is considered. For example, it has been known for 200 years or more that children who are strabismic throughout the first years of life are likely to develop amblyopia. Our own studies on congenital strabismics will be discussed below. The devastating effects on visual development of unoperated bilateral congenital cataract have also been known for many years. This condition will also be discussed below. The effects of extra visual input are hard to quantify, given that in normal children it is difficult to decide what is meant by 'extra' and in cases of visual disability, where extra visual stimulation is given as part of therapy, there are complex interactions between visual disabilities and additional disabilities which make it hard to measure the efficacy of treatment in the visual domain in isolation. Below, some of our own studies on extra stimulation are considered along with situations in which visual input has been reduced because of a clinical condition.

9.1.1 What are the effects of extra visual stimulation in normal children on visual brain development?

Two conditions studied in our unit are:

1. Neurologically normal, very low birth weight (VLBW) premature infants with extra visual experience due to being born earlier than normal.
2. Two normal term infants with enhanced exposure to particular oblique orientations in early infancy.

9.1.1.1 *Neurologically normal very low birth weight premature infants with extra visual experience.*

The question of the effect of extra visual stimulation is a very difficult one in that there has never been a human study comparing matched groups of normal term infants, where the amount and type of visual stimulation has been systematically varied across groups and the groups' visual outcomes compared. Indeed it would probably be very difficult ethically to carry out such a study.

However, a naturally occurring human experiment is the case of healthy premature babies, who often have a month or more of extra visual experience after birth compared with infants born at term. A number of early studies testing acuity in premature infants suggested either no difference, or at best, a very small gain in visual acuity in the premature group, when they were compared with a group of infants born at term (e.g. van Hof-van Duin *et al.* 1989). When carrying out these comparisons of premature and normal infants born at term, the age is calculated from the expected term date rather than the actual date of birth. This is referred to either as matching the *post-conceptual age* or the *post-term age*. These results suggested that much of very early visual development was not affected by extra visual experience.

In our own studies visual development was looked at in a group of premature infants, matched in post-term age to infants born at term, taken from the same postnatal hospital wards. Extensive testing for behavioural and visual evoked potential (VEP) markers of development was included, such as the orientation-reversal VEPs (see Chapter 6) and the ABCDEFV test battery (see Chapter 2).

Initial results suggested that the cohort of premature infants taken as a whole appear to have on average smaller amplitude orientation-reversal VEPs than the mean for the control group and that some of these premature infants are late in age to show a significant orientation-reversal VEP response, compared with the term infant controls. This may indicate that development of the cortex is delayed in these premature infants (see Fig. 9.1).

The premature infants all had a standard examination using ultrasound, to detect

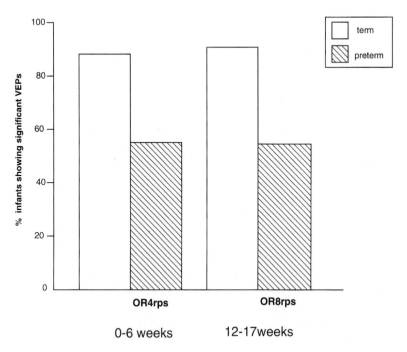

Fig. 9.1 Comparison data on orientation VEPs for the entire premature group of infants and the group of term infants. Note that it appears that the premature group are delayed in development compared with the term infants.

structural brain damage. If we take out of the premature cohort any child who from ultrasound results showed an abnormality which would be suggestive of fetal or peri-natal brain damage, and now compare the two groups (premature and term controls, matched for post-term age), these differences, in onset time for a significant orienta-tion reversal VEP, disappear (Fig. 9.2). This means that the premature infants, with normal ultrasound scans, who were also normal on early neurological tests, develop these responses of cortical function when they are the same *post-term* (conceptual) age as term infants. Of course, this result also suggests that the extra visual stimulation, received by the premature infants, has not accelerated development of the visual cor-tex in these children.

There are several cautionary notes needed here. First, it is not known whether the fact that many of these infants had much of their extra visual experience in an incu-bator means that they had *abnormal* extra visual experience rather than *normal*. There has been much discussion of the effects of high light levels in neonatal intensive care units (for review see Fielder *et al.* 1993). Secondly, the whole idea of starting from a normal baseline for premature infants must be questioned. For many of these infants there are precipitating events related to premature birth which may affect development. Thirdly, the VEP measure used may just not be sensitive enough to pick up small individual differences in development. Perhaps if it had been feasible

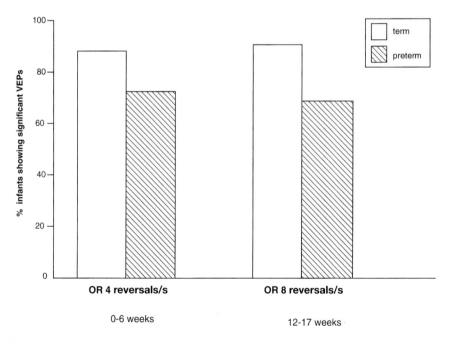

Fig. 9.2 Comparison data on orientation VEPs for the subset of the premature infant group who showed normal ultrasound and the group of term infants (matched controls). Note that there is no significant difference in terms of onset of this cortical VEP between the two groups.

to test these infants at exactly the same time of day and in the same state at weekly intervals it would have been possible to see and measure periods of acceleration in healthy premature infants related to their extra visual stimulation. Of course, sceptics would then have argued that it wasn't the additional visual experience leading to accelerated development, but rather to the intrinsic genetically programmed developmental qualities of premature infants—the 'premature superbabe' theory, by which some have argued that many healthy premature babies are born early because their development all through fetal life has been accelerated.

One of the early behavioural measures of visual development, made at about 4–6 weeks post-term age, did show a brief acceleration in development for the premature infants compared with term infants. This was in measures of saccadic shifts as indicators of shifts of attention between a centrally fixated target and a target which appeared in the periphery (see discussion of the fixation shift measure of attention in Chapter 8). Although there was no difference in the number of correct refixations between the premature infants and term infants, the mean latency for making a saccadic shift was significantly shorter for the premature than the term infants (in both experimental conditions—the *non-competition* condition in which the central target disappears when the peripheral target appears, and the *competition* condition where the central target remains visible when the peripheral target appears). As has already been argued in the discussion on attentional development (Chapter 8), the ability to disengage attention from one target to another while both targets are still visible requires cortical functioning. It follows from this argument that differential performance between the premature and term infants on the competition condition, alone, would indicate accelerated cortical functioning. This is not what is found. It may be that the shorter latencies in both competition and non-competition conditions for the premature group represent a possible acceleration in motor control (in terms of head and eye movements) rather than accelerated cortical development of circuits for selective attention. There is another possibility here and that is the 'premature superbabe theory' mentioned above. This argument would be that premature infants are premature because there are genetic factors either within the fetus or the maternal/fetus interaction, which not only cause more rapid development *in utero*, but also more rapid development postnatally, than in term babies. Perhaps some of our premature infants in this study are 'superbabes' rather than infants where it was necessary to be born early to avoid disastrous consequences. The shortened latency in making saccadic shifts to a peripheral target may be a manifestation of their more rapid development in terms of eye movements generally. Alternatively, it could be that this measure is much more dependent on attentional state than many of our other measures, and these premature infants are less labile in terms of state than normal term infants at 1 month of post-term age. Further tests are needed to distinguish these possibilities.

When comparing other behavioural measures of visual maturity between the entire group of healthy prematures, and the control term infants, it was found that there were no significant differences in their acuity measured using forced-choice preferential looking (FPL) at either 2–3 months of age (mean acuity premature = 3.8 cycles/degree, term = 5.3 cycles/degree) or 7 months of age (mean acuity premature

= 5.6 cycles/degree, term = 6.7 cycles/degree), in the age at which they showed symmetrical monocular optokinetic nystagmus (OKN) responses (between 2 and 4 months), or in their accommodative ability and cycloplegic refraction at 7 months of age (measured using videorefraction). However, on the entire ABCDEFV battery (see Chapter 2), carried out at 4–6 months post-term age, it was found that there were significantly more failures in the premature group than in the control term group. This was largely because of multiple failures by the subset of premature infants who had evidence of brain damage on ultrasound. Again, when the infants who had marked ultrasound abnormalities were taken out and the remaining premature group was compared with controls, there was no significant difference between them; however, there was still a tendency for there to be slightly more failures in the healthy premature group than in the term group.

The main conclusion from this series of studies is that there is no clear evidence of lasting accelerated visual development in the premature group either due to additional visual stimulation or on the basis of them being 'superbabes', with one exception. This was the isolated result that the premature group showed slightly quicker mean saccadic responses in terms of lateral orienting to a peripheral target in the fixation shift test compared with the term infants, at about 1 month post-term age.

9.1.1.2 *Two infants with enhanced exposure to particular oblique orientations in early infancy*

There is a good deal of evidence that early experience with oriented contours can affect the distribution of orientation-selective neurons in the cortex (Blakemore and Cooper 1970; Hirsch and Spinelli 1970; Stryker *et al.* 1978; Rauschecker and Singer 1981). The well known *'oblique effect'* is the higher resolution acuity for lines oriented along the vertical and horizontal meridians compared with lines obliquely orientated (Appelle 1972). It is considered to be the result of enhanced neuronal representation within the cortex for lines oriented along the major meridians because of extensive exposure to these orientations, rather than oblique retinal orientations, throughout early life (Mitchell *et al.* 1973). There has been some dispute concerning the argument made for the so-called 'carpentered environment'—that is the idea that the visual world for babies living in a man-made environment contains a bias in exposure to vertical and horizontal lines produced by the boundaries between walls in rooms. The debate concerns whether a real bias in retinal orientation exposure exists in everyday life. Nevertheless, the *oblique effect* is found to a varying extent in most adults with normal vision.

To see whether enhanced exposure to obliquely oriented lines in infancy affected the adult acuity in different meridians, and could be an environmental procedure to negate the oblique effect, Fleur, our oldest daughter, had an enriched environment in terms of oblique orientations. Her cot bumpers in her carrycot, crib, and pram had patterned covers made up of obliquely oriented lines (in terms of retinal stimulation if she was lying with her head on one side). She was exposed to these patterns for a period from 3 weeks post-term age to 8 months of age. These cushions were especially constructed to contain a variety of stripe widths and colours across a wide range of spatial frequencies against a white background. Ione (our youngest child) had a somewhat different type of enhanced stimulation with obliquely oriented lines. She was tested in approximately 150 separate sessions (each 10–45 min in length) between day 1 and 3.5 months of age, for multiple measures of contrast sensitivity, acuity, and orientation reversal VEPs (OR-VEPs) (see Chapter 4 and Atkinson and Braddick, 1989, for details of this study). All stimuli in these testing sessions were obliquely oriented grating patterns, varying in contrast and spatial frequency. We estimated that this exposure for both Fleur and Ione was between 5 and 10% of their waking time at this young age. Both children were later tested with Keeler acuity cards, with the cards rotated in the vertical, horizontal, and 45° orientation for the stripes (Atkinson *et al.* 1992*b*). Fleur was tested at 18 years (wearing a small refractive correction for myopic astigmatism) and Ione at 3.2 years. Lorrin (brother of Ione and Fleur) who did not have any special exposure in infancy was tested using the same procedure. Ione and Lorrin had not had significant refractive errors at any stage of development.

The Keeler cards were selected because they present gratings in a circular 'window'. However, a thin white annulus separates the gratings from the grey background, and the ends of the grating bars form a detectably 'jagged' edge. This acuity measure may, therefore, reflect performance on a vernier cue, explaining the high values sometimes obtained, especially in older subjects.

The oblique effect was measured as a ratio of acuity estimate for the obliquely oriented lines compared with the vertically or horizontally oriented lines. Fleur and Ione have had extra visual experience, early in life, with obliquely oriented grating patterns. The histogram shows a comparison of the grating acuities for all three children, for lines vertically, horizontally and obliquely oriented. As can be seen from Fig. 9.3, all three children showed very similar levels of the oblique effect (acuity for oblique 70–80% that for the mean of the horizontal and vertical), and levels that are close to the published adult norms. There was no indication that the biasing of the developing systems had been altered by enhanced exposure to the obliquely oriented lines.

The conclusions from our own limited studies on extra visual experience in infancy would suggest one of two things. One is that there is little possibility of accelerating development of some parts of the visual system in the first few months of life, including accelerating the orientation tuning and onset of cortical systems for discriminating orientation by providing extra pattern stimulation. Alternatively, it could be argued that the extra visual stimulation which has been given in these studies is very minimal and is not great enough to accelerate the early processes of cortical functioning. It is quite possible that the system for orientation sensitivity in the early stages of cortical onset is not a particularly plastic one. This is supported by data from studies by Mike Stryker and his colleagues, who have found that the arrangement of orientation columns appears to be pre-programmed and unchanged by early monocular deprivation (Crair *et al.* 1998).

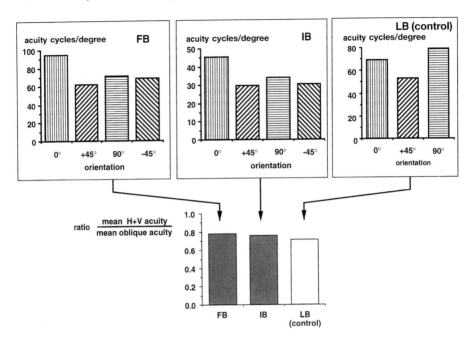

Fig. 9.3 Oblique effect in Fleur, Ione, and Lorrin.

9.1.2 What are the effects of reduced or anomalous visual input on visual brain development?

Three conditions that we have studied will be considered here.

1. Effects of reduced input due to congenital bilateral cataract.
2. Effects of anomalous input due to congenital strabismus, followed by relatively early surgery.
3. Effects of degraded input due to refractive errors (e.g. anisometropia, astigmatism) in early infancy.

All of these conditions are associated with the development of amblyopia. Amblyopia is defined as a deficit in visual acuity, that is not correctable by spectacles, and not associated with visible pathology of the eye. The deficit continues even if the original condition is corrected, because the eye has become functionally ineffective in its connections to the cortex. Most commonly, this is a functional loss for one eye, resulting from competitive interactions with the other eye in establishing cortical connections.

Although amblyopia is clinically defined in terms of acuity, it is clear that at least some amblyopia (especially strabismic amblyopia) involves deficits of perception that go beyond a simple loss of resolution. Patterns may appear to be scrambled or distorted (e.g. see Hess, Campbell and Greenhalgh 1978). These effects have not yet been at all thoroughly investigated in children. However, acuity measures such as Snellen charts, but not simple grating acuity, do reflect in part these 'scrambling' effects, which are also described as 'crowding' by the adjacent letters in the chart. We have devised and used 'crowding cards' (Chapter 2) as an acuity test which reflects the full amblyopic deficit, and which children can perform before they are capable of reading a Snellen chart. Many of our results to be described use this approach.

9.1.2.1 *Effects of congenital cataract and strabismus on development*

9.1.2.1.1 Congenital cataract

Our first clinical case of congenital cataract, seen in 1978, was a neurologically normal child, born with congenital bilateral cataracts and operated on at 2 weeks of age in one eye and 3 weeks of age in the second eye (patient SJ). The measurements of his acuity immediately after successful surgery, and development following surgery, are shown in Fig. 9.4, together with comparable measurements from cross-sectional data in groups of normal infants with the same FPL set-up, collected in our lab at the same time. As can be seen, SJ makes an excellent start in terms of catching up on the normal trajectory for acuity, but persistently falls short of the norms beyond 2 years of age. One complication is that many of these children, including SJ, develop strabismus and have congenital early-onset nystagmus. These factors in themselves will alter visual development. Extensive longitudinal studies of cataract, surgery, and occlusion therapy have been carried out (e.g. Birch *et al.* 1986; Maurer and Lewis 1993). The general finding seems to be that deprivation from 3 to 18 months often has a marked effect, but that spectacle or interocular lens implant plus occlusion therapy during this period can markedly reduce the density of amblyopia. An additional interesting finding is that there are very rapid rises in acuity in the first hours after surgical recovery and corrective lens placement (Maurer *et al.* 1999).

Deprivation in one eye by monocular cataract creates amblyopia due to interocular competition in development. Occlusion therapy attempts to alleviate this competition by periods in which the 'good eye' is covered. The goal is to minimize unilateral amblyopia while also minimalizing any possibility of reverse amblyopia in the patched 'good' eye. Extensive primate studies of different occlusion regimens suggest that there is an optimal level for occlusion therapy of about 70% of waking time within the critical period, for monocular occlusion of the good eye to bring about the optimal levels of acuity in both eyes as the final outcome in adulthood (for review see Boothe 1996). It is not known whether this is also the optimum treatment strategy in human infants, although from the extensive studies that have been completed so far, the general consensus is that great care must be taken in the first year of life with the extent of monocular occlusion therapy, to reduce the possibility of reverse amblyopia being induced in the 'good' patched eye. However, many clinicians believe that in cases of unilateral cataract, relatively aggressive continuous occlusion of the good eye in the first years of life following surgery and correcting lenses is a necessity, if vision in the poor eye is to be able to develop. The decision on occlusion

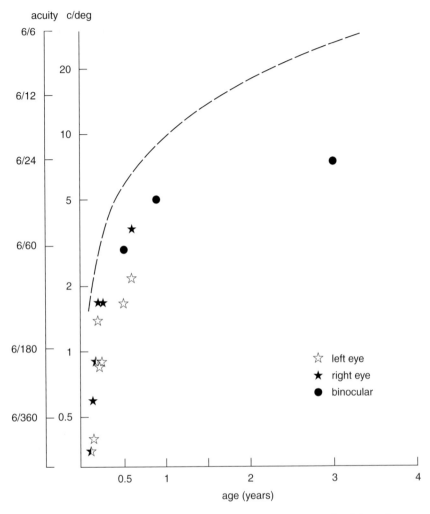

Fig. 9.4 Development of visual acuity following early surgery for bilateral congenital cataract.

therapy in monocular cataract is a very difficult one, clinically and ethically. To maintain a child in a regimen of unilateral occlusion of the good eye, and thus to prevent optimal monocular vision throughout an extended period of development, so that some development may be achieved in an eye which has started life with a defect, is an extremely difficult decision and an arduous task for parents.

9.1.2.1.2 Early-onset strabismus

Chapter 6 has described the correlogram and stereogram stimuli used to test whether the infant was combining information from the two eyes' images to detect binocular correlation and binocular disparity. Using these stimuli it has been seen that in normal development information is combined between the eyes at about 3–4 months of post-term age. Here we consider what happens when development of binocularity is abnormal in what is called 'early-onset' or 'congenital' strabismus. The term 'congenital' may be misleading if it is taken to imply that the child is born with a defect of cortical binocularity. It might be preferable to call it 'early-onset' strabismus in that the problem may not be in disparity-detection mechanisms as such. Problems in setting up disparity tuning may be a consequence of a preceding faulty mechanism, such as the alignment mechanism of the eyes in convergence.

There is ample evidence, from animal physiology and clinical experience, that the binocular organization of visual cortex remains highly modifiable for a period after it is initially established (see review by Daw 1995). The maintenance of binocular function depends on a critical synergy between mechanisms that detect binocular relationships in the images from the two eyes, and the motor mechanisms that control alignment. Accurate vergence control depends on disparity-sensitive mechanisms to provide the main controlling input; but disparity-sensitive mechanisms can be degraded or destroyed if they do not receive the correlated inputs provided by well-aligned eyes. The high incidence of strabismus in all paediatric neurological conditions (see, for example, Atkinson and van Hof-van Duin 1993) shows that this loop is fragile and readily broken.

Chapter 6 has already discussed whether the visual experience associated with well aligned eyes is necessary for the initial establishment of cortical binocularity. The conclusions from the studies of Birch and Stager (1985; Birch 1993) on infants with early esotropia, would suggest that this was not so. They carried out longitudinal studies with infants with early esotropia, wearing prisms to compensate for the angle of deviation, and found that up to 4 months, the proportion of esotropic infants showing disparity sensitivity was similar to that of a normal group. However, beyond this age, the number giving positive results increased in the normal group but steeply declined among the esotropes. It seems that aligned binocular input was necessary to sustain binocular mechanisms in this group, even though it was not a necessary prerequisite.

Birch and Stager's result also implies that an absence of sensory binocularity did not generally cause the early-onset strabismus. This is consistent with the results of a study in our Unit (Wattam-Bell *et al.* 1987) which followed a group of infants whose family history put them at risk for strabismus. Among this group were infants who showed positive responses on the correlogram VEP test between 11 and 20 weeks, but developed manifest strabismus after this age and before 6 months of age. The results of both studies suggest that the sensory-motor loop was initially disrupted on the motor rather than the sensory side. This is not to deny of course, the existence of conditions where a failure of sensory binocularity is primary, for example where the visual pathways are congenitally misrouted as in ocular albinism (Apkarian 1996; Guillery 1996).

If an infant's eyes are misaligned initially then is it at all possible for them to set up binocular interactions between points in the two eyes' fields that correspond to the angle of misalignment or deviation? In other words, are there limits to the plasticity of the binocular system so that the eyes have to be aligned within a certain range for these binocular correlations to be set up? Data from our studies on a group of children with onset of strabismus in the first year and surgery before the age of 2 years, suggest quite extensive ranges of plasticity in some children (Smith *et al.* 1991). Disparity selectivity was measured before and after surgery, and it was found that infants who showed a strongly preferred eye for fixation generally gave negative results pre-operatively in FPL disparity testing. However, among the children who could fixate with either eye pre-operatively, the majority showed responses to a stereo disparity of 40 min (a relatively large disparity) before surgery. There was no prism correction for the deviation during these tests, so these results imply binocular inter-actions corresponding to the angle of deviation, which was typically about 30 prism dioptres. This suggests extensive early plasticity in setting up disparity tuning in the first year of life. Following surgical correction (and therapy), many of the group gave positive results on the FPL stereo test. This implies that at the age of surgery (11–27 months) the system is sufficiently plastic to re-establish binocular interactions between the newly aligned corresponding points. However, this appears to be a tran-sient effect. Many of these children at age 4 years were re-examined, with a variety of stereo tests. There was essentially no evidence of persisting stereopsis, even on the FPL test for which the same children had shown positive responses about 2 years ear-lier. A similar conclusion was reached by Charles and Moore (1992) from clinic follow-up of an extended study of the same group of children. The reasons for the failure to maintain binocularity are unclear: possibly the re-established or modified binocular-ity is weak or fragmentary, and so is vulnerable to disruptions of sensory-motor syn-ergy which a better-established system could withstand; possibly the forces leading to the original strabismus persist, although the surgical and orthoptic therapy may mean that their oculomotor consequences are less easily detectable.

9.1.2.1.3 Accommodative esotropia

A more subtly disrupting condition, which may lead to esotropia, is the stress on the accommodation–convergence relationship caused by marked hyperopic refractive error. The concept of accommodative esotropia has arisen from the hyperopic refrac-tive errors found in children at the time they present to the clinician with strabis-mus. The photo- and videorefractive screening programmes (discussed briefly in Chapter 5) indicated the links between hyperopia and strabismus. However, the detailed dynamics by which hyperopia leads to a disruption of the sensory-motor binocular loop are still only poorly understood. The general idea is that hyperopic infants need to make a larger amount of accommodation than emmetropic infants, and that because of the natural synergy between accommodation and convergence, the extra accommodation leads to overconvergence which becomes manifested as esotropia. The theory assumes a relationship between the degree of accommodation and convergence (measured as the AC/A ratio), but does not give any explanation as to why this ratio cannot be adapted appropriately in cases of infant hyperopia.

In our first screening programme it was found that there was a positive correla-tion between infants who were markedly hyperopic under cycloplegia and those who became strabismic. However, by no means all infants with hyperopia became strabismic. This suggests that there must be an additional factor to explain the individual variations in vulnerability to strabismus of infants with hyperopic refractions. It was also found in the first screening programme that hyperopic infants varied in the extent to which they adequately accommodated for nearby targets. In fact many were extremely poor accommodators throughout infancy. Such behaviour would suggest that their esotropia was unlikely to be due to excessive accommodation and a breakdown in convergence. In the second, current infant screening programme, accommodative performance without cycloplegia forms the screening measure (see Atkinson *et al*. 1996). Infants who were poor accommodators were selected at screening and followed up to see whether they have marked hyperopia under cycloplegia. Many of them do, although there is an interesting group whose degree of accommodative lag without cycloplegia is almost identical to their hyperopic refractive error. There is an additional small group who appear to accommodate well on screening, and were among the control group, but who show marked hyperopia under cycloplegia at first follow-up. On the basis of the theory of accommodative esotropia, these later infants should perhaps be at great risk of strabismus. So far, there is rather little evidence that this group are at any higher risk of strabismus than the poor accomodators. The final visual outcome of these infants, identified with marked hyperopia in infancy from this programme, may help to identify the interactions of accommodation with refraction that create the high likelihood of strabismus in some hyperopic infants but not others, and the relationship between accommodative performance and refractive error throughout infancy.

9.1.2.1.4 Underlying physiology of early binocular plasticity

The classic studies of the cat by Wiesel and Hubel (1963) showed that closure of one eye in kittens caused marked changes in the structure and function of the visual pathways. The closed eye became amblyopic and much less effective in driving cells in the visual cortex. Neuronal cell bodies in the lateral geniculate nucleus (LGN) laminae related to the closed eye appeared smaller when compared with those from the open eye. In fact the difference of size has been found to be due to hypertrophy of the undeprived cells rather than shrinkage of deprived cells (Sloper 1993). These effects were only seen if the monocular deprivation was in the first months of life and was much greater if one eye was closed than if both were closed in this early period. This suggested that the effects were due in part to competitive processes between the pathways related to the two eyes. During this early period the ocular dominance columns within the cortex segregate for each eye and there will be changes in width depending on the extent of monocular deprivation If monocular deprivation starts much later, i.e. after the first few months of life, a second sensitive period can be delineated in primates which is characterized by shrinkage of cells in both deprived and undeprived LGN layers, specifically in the parvocellular layers rather than both magnocellular and parvocellular layers. In primates this latter sensitive period extends from about 8 weeks of age to 1 year (Sloper 1993). During this period the predominant interaction between the pathways to the two eyes is cooperative and hence has little effect on the relative width of ocular dominance columns in layer IV, which is the monocular input layer of cortex. However, late monocular deprivation has been shown to affect deeper and more superficial layers outside layer IV, where binocular interactions first occur. As these interactions depend on inputs from the two eyes, if one eye is deprived then input from neither eye can be used in this way, and the shrinkage of both eye's input cells may reflect this lack of binocularity.

Unfortunately, little is known about the timing of ocular dominance segregation within the human cortex. In a preliminary report Hickey and Peduzzi (1987) found well-formed columns in a human 6 month old and poorly formed columns in a 4 month old. This result fits quite well with the idea that ocular segregation probably occurs at approximately the same time as onset of stereopsis in humans. From models of stereopsis developed in Sejnowski's group, there has been the suggestion that binocular co-ordination of the signals between cells is necessary before cells sensitive to disparity develop (Berns *et al.* 1993). If there is correlation within each eye's signals, but not correlation between eyes then only monocular cells develop. If there is a two-stage process with correlation within each eye preceding correlation between eyes the model produces binocular cells sensitive to zero disparity and monocular cells sensitive to non-zero disparity.

There are now extensive cat and primate studies looking at the neurochemical factors and cellular mechanisms by which plasticity for binocular interactions is reduced or enhanced. A good review is given in Daw (1995, chapter 12) For example, it has been found that the concentration of N-methyl-D-aspartate (NMDA) receptors correlates well with the peak of the sensitive period in cat, and this is also correlated with calcium levels. Levels of protein kinase C found in the visual cortex, also follows the time factors of the critical period. It is well known from a number of studies that dark rearing can delay the onset of the critical period. Dark rearing also postpones the reduction in NMDA contribution to the visual response and thus makes these links to plasticity more plausible. However, most of these links have yet to be worked out in the case of human development.

Overall, it is clear that the cortical interaction of signals from the two eyes is a highly plastic system in early life. There are a number of different levels at which this plasticity occurs, and plasticity beyond the level of primary visual cortex (V1) has been very little explored. The function of this plasticity, presumably, is to tune the interacting combination of neural, optical, and oculomotor systems in the growing child, to achieve a level of precision in binocular vision that could not be attained by a more rigid pattern of development. However, there are clearly strong constraints on this plasticity, both in the level of mismatch between these systems that can be successfully adjusted, and in the period of development over which adjustment can take place.

9.1.3.1 *Effects of reduced input due to refractive errors, e.g. children with a history of refractive errors (e.g. anisometropia, astigmatism) identified, but not corrected, in infancy*

It is well known that extended periods of optical blur, due to errors of focus, lead to changes in the cortical systems which can be measured psychophysically as amblyopia.

In particular, both uncorrected anisometropia, and high levels of astigmatism early in life, have been found to be related to amblyopia. However, we know from our screening programmes (described in Chapter 5) that small degrees of anisometropia and quite high levels of astigmatism are quite frequent in normal infant populations, and yet the level of amblyopia is far lower in normal adult populations (2–5% dependent on criteria, method of measurement, and study population). This means that the majority of children must lose these refractive errors in time for natural plasticity to allow the cortical visual system to be modified to give normal adult vision without amblyopia. There is of course the argument that nearly all of us, at least all adults who show an oblique effect, may have a mild form of meridional amblyopia. That is, that the poorer acuity for oblique lines compared with vertical and horizontal lines is the remaining effect in adulthood of defocus due to astigmatism in early infancy (astigmatism with a horizontal or vertical axis showing the greater defocus will mean that at different times, horizontal or vertical contours, but never obliques, can be brought into good focus). To support this hypothesis, there would need to be data comparing or correlating the degree of infant astigmatism in individuals to the size of their later oblique effect; these data do not seem to be available at present.

In Chapter 5 a little was said about our screening programmes and the results which bear directly on the question of the effect of early refractive errors on later visual development. In the first photorefractive screening programme, a randomized control trial was run in which spectacles were given (to obtain a partial correction of refractive errors) to half the hyperopic infant population. In this trial, not all of the children offered spectacles consistently wore their correction and so these children can be considered *untreated* in terms of refractive error. The formula for deciding the appropriate spectacle correction, offered in the randomized trial, was conservative and so did not attempt to correct all the hyperopia or astigmatism. This conservatism was due to our knowledge of infant astigmatism and its changes with age. In a previous study where levels of astigmatism were measured longitudinally in individual infants, it was found that most astigmatic infants showed reduction in astigmatism between 3 and 24 months of age (Atkinson *et al.* 1980). Because of our knowledge of this naturally occurring process of normalization (*emmetropization*), it was decided that we must be careful not to give an astigmatic correction which would risk overcorrecting the astigmatic component if the child wore the same correction for several months between their refractive assessments. Consequently, most of the corrections given were largely for the spherical component of their refractive error and not for the cylindrical component (astigmatism). This means that it is possible that some of the corrected spectacle wearers were still mildly optically defocused due to astigmatic errors. The other point to remember is that in the first programme, all refractive errors were measured at screening under cycloplegia and the exact amount of optical blur experienced in everyday life was likely to be less, because of attempts made to accommodate to some extent by most infants (even those with hyperopic refractive errors). However, although most infant hyperopes accommodate to some extent, many do not maintain accommodation consistently. Again, this variability of accommodation both within and between infants, will tend to make the data more noisy.

However, given these caveats, we found major differences in visual outcome between the group of infants who had been significantly hyperopic and worn spectacles to correct partially their refractive error, the group of hyperopic infants who had not worn a correction, and the control group who were normal refractively at screening. The untreated hyperopes were 13 times more likely than controls to develop strabismus by 4 years of age (21% of untreated hyperopes), whereas the treated group showed a much lower incidence of strabismus (6.3%) which was higher but not significantly different in incidence of strabismus to the control group (1.6%). Secondly, the group of infants who showed marked hyperopic refractive errors in infancy and who did not wear a spectacle correction, were significantly more likely to have poor acuity than both those who wore spectacles and the normal control infants (who were emmetropic at screening). This poor acuity was identified using the Cambridge Crowding Cards. However, recognition of letter targets could be impaired by poor acuity in any meridian. This is called *meridional amblyopia* (see Mitchell *et al.* 1973; Gwiazda *et al.* 1986). To examine this possibility, a subset of the untreated hyperopic group was tested for meridional amblyopia with grating stimuli in different meridians, using an automated FPL procedure when they were 4 years of age (Atkinson *et al.* 1982). Of course, at the time of testing any residual refractive errors were corrected so that any reduction in acuity could not be the direct result of refractive blur. Acuity measures were taken for vertically and horizontally oriented sinusoidal grating patterns. If a reliable difference of more than 0.67 octaves was found between acuity in the two meridians, the child was deemed to be showing some meridional amblyopia.

The refractive changes over the course of the first 3 years were examined in the same children (who had been infant hyperopes at screening) and the group was divided into those who were persistently astigmatic (over 1 D) after 2 years of age, and those who had lost their astigmatism by 2 years. As can be seen in Fig. 9.5, there is a strong relationship between those showing meridional amblyopia (as measured in the modified FPL test), and persistence of astigmatism beyond 2 years. Measures of meridional amblyopia were also compared with the same child's performance on the Cambridge Crowding Cards acuity test at 4 years (Fig. 9.6).

Children who failed the acuity tests tended also to be those who showed meridional amblyopia. However, there is a significant group who failed the letter test but were not deemed meridional amblyopes on this criterion using the results of the FPL grating test. It has been pointed out earlier that grating acuity does not necessarily reflect the 'scrambling' effects reported in amblyopia. A scrambled perception could still allow grating orientation to be successfully recognized; the requirement to recognize and distinguish letter shapes in the Crowding Cards is a more sensitive test of amblyopia. One possibility, therefore, is that some of the uncorrected hyperopes were mildly amblyopic, not enough to show marked relative reductions in grating acuity, but enough to show reduced acuity on the Crowding Cards. The other possibility is that the Crowding Cards, with the need to maintain attention on the concept of the 'middle' letter, place an additional cognitive demand. It may be that children who still showed reduced acuity on the letter matching test at 4 years, but were not children who had persistent astigmatism beyond 2 years of age, are showing small global lags in all aspects of visuocognitive development. From the first

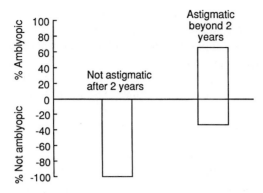

Fig. 9.5 Relationship between meridional amblyopia and persistence of astigmatism beyond 2 years of age.

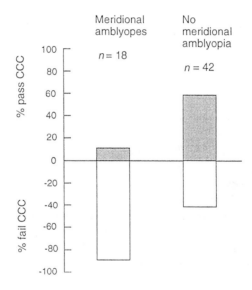

Fig. 9.6 Crowding Cards (CCC) test results compared with meridional amblyopia.

screening programme these factors cannot be separated out, but in the second screening programme, where more extensive visuocognitive measures are used at 4–6 years, we may be able to attempt to answer this question in the future.

From the results so far we believe that spectacle wear (to correct hyperopic refractive errors, including astigmatic errors) can be a successful treatment for many children with hyperopic refractive errors in infancy to prevent amblyopia in the pre-school years.

Although these screening outcome data show that the sensitivity of the developing cortical system to different orientations can be modified by the optical input throughout infancy, the results do not suggest whether there is any remaining plasticity beyond 4 years. One problem here is to decide whether there is any appropriate treatment for those who appear to show meridional amblyopia at 4 years, but who do not require any correction for astigmatism by this age (their large levels of infant astigmatism having reduced between 2 and 4 years). This was the case for many of these children in the first screening programme who had lost much of their hyperopia and astigmatism by 4 years of age. In the second screening programme amblyopia has been measured at 3.5–6 years to gauge the extent of this critical period of later development.

Another line of evidence on the onset of amblyopia comes from the study of congenitally esotropic children. Birch and Stager (1985) measured the acuity of each eye at different ages. As interocular acuity differences can be found in normal young infants (Atkinson *et al.* 1982) it is often difficult to quantify the extent of amblyopia in congenital esotropes. However, Birch and Stager reported that the interocular difference in esotropic infants did not go outside the normal range until 9–11 months of age. This result suggests that strabismus in the first year of life does not lead to amblyopia, analogous to our findings above, which suggest that refractive errors over the same period do not generally lead to amblyopia. It is only if these refractive errors persist beyond 2 years of age that there is a high risk of amblyopia.

9.2 DOES ABNORMAL INPUT PRODUCE CHANGES IN MORE PERIPHERAL VISUAL SYSTEMS?

9.2.1 Deprivation myopia and emmetropization

Chapter 5 discussed data on emmetropization from the Cambridge Infant screening programmes; emmetropization is the process whereby the eyeball grows in most infants to be the correct size in adulthood for the image to be in focus on the retina. Most infants are born slightly hyperopic in terms of refractive state, although they normally take up a somewhat myopic focus when actively accommodating. Most infants become emmetropic by 3 years of age and some become more myopic after 4–5 years, leading to between 10 and 50% adult myopes (there are considerable differences between populations, including racial differences). In these cases the eyeball has grown too large for the power of the lens and cornea. Very few infants showed large myopic refractive errors in infancy and those with small degrees of myopia tended to emmetropize initially before 4 years.

It has been well known for some time (one of the first studies being by Wiesel and Raviola 1977) that in many species, including humans, monocular deprivation of pattern vision causes not only central changes but also a tendency to myopia. For example, in one study by Johnson *et al.* (1982) the refraction of twins was compared, one of each twin having a congenital lens opacity in one eye. The affected eye was found to be 2 mm longer than the unaffected, whereas very small differences were found in the members of the twin pairs who did not have the early deprivation.

In the case of complete opacity the results are reasonably consistent from one study to another, the general conclusion being that visual feedback is necessary for the growth of the lens, cornea, and eyeball to keep in step to achieve emmetropization. However, there is some debate about the range and magnitude of the compensation due to optical feedback (for example, see Schaeffel 1993; Hung *et al.* 1995). As part of our screening programme, including the randomized control trial, the first comparison of human emmetropization in infants was carried out, matched for refractive errors in infancy, with one group wearing a spectacle correction for their hyperopic refractive errors and the other group uncorrected. An important point, already made in the discussion of astigmatism above, is that the correction prescribed in the screening programme was conservative to avoid the overcorrection of reducing refractive errors. With the partial correction, these infants would have to make less accommodative effort to achieve a focused image, but some accommodation would still be necessary.

Chapter 5 has already discussed refractive changes found in different groups in the first screening programme. For the control group, emmetropization consisted of a small reduction in the level of astigmatism in the first 2 years of life. A similar result has been found in the second screening programme (Ehrlich *et al.* 1995, 1996).

When hyperopic infants wearing a refractive correction were compared with those who were not wearing spectacles, no significant differences in their rate of emmetropization were found. It does not seem that the partial spectacle correction is preventing emmetropization in this case. However, a significant finding here is that both the hyperopic groups are still more hyperopic at 3 years than the control infants, and have not emmetropized to normal adult levels. Whether they ever do, remains an open question. We hope to follow these children up to 6 years in our second screening programme to see whether they remain significantly hyperopic or reduce to emmetropia at a later age than the controls. These data support the idea that emmetropization has not been affected by partial correction. It could be that the factors controlling human emmetropization, compared with other species, do not involve very great plasticity, in order that relatively small refractive errors in infancy do not trigger rapid changes which would then need to be reversed at a later stage.

In the screening study, most hyperopic refractive errors were between 3 and 5 D and given spectacle corrections between 2 and 4 D: these may not be of sufficient magnitude to alter the normal course of emmetropization. It is quite possible that the use of full, rather than partial, correction could have disrupted emmetropization because this would have negated completely the signal from optical blur. This would not be in agreement with the results of Hung *et al.* (1995) in monkeys. This group found compensation for small amounts of refractive anisometropia but anomalous results for −10 D lenses where a smaller rather than larger eyeball was found. It is possible that the system treats the lack of a well formed image as myopia, and then compensates by reduces eye growth leading to hyperopia (Kiorpes and Wallman 1995). Certainly we have no documented cases of large hyperopic refractive corrections leading to marked hyperopia rather than myopia. The true differences between the extent of plasticity in humans and other primates, if they exist, remains to be evaluated.

A remaining question is why there are very large individual differences in the rate of emmetropization in the hyperopic infants. The retinal mechanisms controlling eye growth are not yet understood, although it is known that major changes associated with eye enlargement are an increase in DNA and protein synthesis and proteoglycan in the sclera (Christensen and Wallman 1991; Rada *et al.* 1991). It seems that the various growth factors controlling these processes have yet to be elucidated. However, it is also known that neural feedback loops are important in the human, and these must interact with local factors in the eye. It seems quite plausible that there may be individual differences in both local growth hormone factors and the efficiency of feedback mechanisms between refractive errors and accommodation. We know that poor emmetropization, leaving marked refractive errors in later childhood, combined with poor accommodation is a widespread finding in all paediatric neurological populations (e.g. in cerebral palsy). It seems quite plausible that similar but much milder deficiencies at the biochemical level could underlie these limitations in plasticity in individual, apparently neurologically normal, infants with marked refractive errors.

9.3 DOES BRAIN DAMAGE OR EARLY ABNORMAL BRAIN STRUCTURE PRODUCE COMPENSATING CHANGES IN VISUAL SYSTEMS?

The previous section discussed compensatory visual development following either changes in environmental factors outside the infant, or in more peripheral mechanisms. Here the mechanism that may compensate for much more radical changes in the developing brain is considered. Children may be born with a brain abnormality either due to embryological processes that take an abnormal developmental route, or to perinatal events that lead to brain damage. Very often it is difficult to separate precisely these two and it is believed that many perinatal problems are part of a long chain of events *in utero*, many of which cannot be identified at present. An estimated 50% of the clinical referrals seen in our unit for assessing potential visual problems have no identified precursors of these problems from the pregnancy or birth history; not knowing the cause of developmental problems remains a perpetual anxiety for many parents of disabled children. Enormous strides in the neonatology of birth asphyxia have been made both from human studies and in animal models (Thoresen *et al.* 1995; Penrice *et al.* 1996), and there may now be therapeutic interventions that can maintain plasticity in the newborn's brain to encourage recovery from these events (e.g. see Edwards *et al.* 1998). One hopeful possibility is the use of a brief cooling regimen that slows metabolism to interrupt the cascade of events leading to cell death following anoxia.

In this section the compensatory changes in three very different clinical groups will be considered.

1. Visual development following hemispherectomy in infancy.
2. Visual development following very early brain lesions monitored by structural magnetic resonance imaging (MRI) both generalized and focal.
3. Visual development in Williams syndrome (WS).

9.3.1 Visual development following hemispherectomy in infancy

Chapter 8 has already discussed attentional deficits in two infants who underwent complete hemispherectomy (one at 5 months and one at 8 months of age) to relieve intractable focal epilepsy (Braddick *et al.* 1992). By comparing their responses in the left and right half of space (the ipsilateral and contralateral visual field) it was possible to show that if two targets were competing for visual attention, one in foveal view and one in the near periphery, the infants only make eye, head, and hand movements to the peripheral target on the side of space controlled by the remaining good hemisphere. Their remaining subcortical visual system (retinocollicular pathways) does not seem to be able to generate attentional shifts without a cortical command. In these studies it appeared that over time there was no improvement in these responses, but rather that the asymmetries seemed to increase rather than decrease.

Chapter 6 considered the systems controlling optokinetic nystagmus, both for monocular and binocular viewing. Again in these hemisphectomized children we have only found OKN generated by movement of a pattern towards the good remaining hemisphere (i.e. right to left movement for the left hemisphere). This result was the same for monocular and binocular viewing suggesting that lack of cortical mechanisms in one hemisphere can affect both the cortical and subcortical control of OKN. Recently we have studied an even younger case of hemispherectomy, where the child was operated on at 2 months of age. The same persistent asymmetry was seen binocularly, although interestingly in monocular viewing it seems that, for a very early time period of development, the isolated subcortical system on the damaged side, could generate OKN for the direction towards the absent cortex, i.e. OKN could be generated for both directions of pattern movement (Morrone *et al.* 1999).

These results on both attentional shifts and OKN imply a lack of plasticity in the ability of the remaining hemisphere to take over control from the damaged side. This is in contrast to some somatosensory and motor results on older hemispherectomized patients who show compensatory function based on ipsilateral connections to the intact hemisphere. Hemispherectomy is a very extreme case of damage, which may in the visual case remove most or all of the pathways on which any recovery of function might be based.

9.3.2 Visual development following very early brain lesions monitored by structural MRI (both general and focal)

In an ongoing programme of the population referred from the Hammersmith Hospital we have seen over 200 children with a range of potential brain abnormalities from very discrete focal lesions on one side, to extensive bilateral damage to all parts of the brain. The latter is often a result of hypoxic–ischaemic encephalopathy (HIE). These children can be classified either according to clinical neurological signs at birth (Sarnat and Sarnat's, 1976, criteria for three bands of HIE according to severity), or in terms of the structural abnormalities seen on MRI. All the infants in our study have had serial scans throughout the first 2 years of life. In general we considered the MRI records from the scans performed in the neonatal period after the end of the first week of life for term infants. However, in some cases we have compared later MRI results with concurrent visual development.

What can be concluded so far concerning plasticity of visual development in these children recovering from deleterious perinatal events? To answer this question a whole set of visual tests have been carried out throughout the first 4 years of these children's lives, with more testing in the first year than subsequent years (for full details of many of these results see, Mercuri *et al.* 1995, 1996*a,b*, 1997*a,b*, 1998).

If a child is born with damage to the visual cortex, can their vision ever develop normally? The answer to this question will depend on three factors: the extent of the damage; the exact location of the damage; and the intrinsic robustness of the child (which is likely to depend on a variety of genetic and environmental factors, many of which we cannot specify at present). In general terms if an infant is classified as having extensive encephalopathy at birth (grade 3 HIE generalized brain damage and a high likelihood of extensive seizures) then the prognosis for visual development is very poor. It is likely that this child will have severe neurological deficits including 'cortical blindness'. Fortunately, very few surviving full-term infants fall within this category. Many are graded as HIE 1 and HIE 2. In general those in HIE 1 develop vision normally (at least on measures made in the first 2 years) and are in the normal range neurologically and paediatrically at 2 years. This is not to say that they are necessarily at the 50th percentiles or better for their age, or that they will not show any mild visuocognitive deficits at a later stage. For infants classified as HIE 2 it is difficult to make an early prognosis of outcome. Approximately half of those in HIE 2 appear to do well in development like the infants in HIE 1, half appear to be delayed in terms of our indicators of cortical onset (orientation VEPs and fixation shifts by 5 months of age), but many show some recovery by 2–3 years of age. It is suspected that many of these children will show minor visual deficits and visuocognitive deficits at a later stage. They may, of course, show minor deficits in other domains as well. We are currently looking at their early linguistic development, which might also show delays in development.

When the extent of focal lesions detected in neonatal structural MRI and their correlation is compared with individual visual measures it has been found that, although in nearly every case the parietal lobe in some part is affected, lesions of cortical areas alone are not well correlated with the extent of the child's visual problems. Other areas, outside classical visual pathways seem to be crucial for a prognosis of normal development, namely, the basal ganglia and cerebellum.

Table 9.1 shows that infants with basal ganglia damage in isolation (detected on structural MRI) can fail many more early visual tests than infants with extensive damage to the classical visual cortex (Mercuri *et al.* 1997). Those with both basal ganglia and cortical damage (seen on MRI) are worse visually than those with damage to either structure alone. It may be that particular parts of certain structures within the basal ganglia (e.g. the caudate) are heavily involved in particular cortical/basal ganglia circuits, essential for normal visual development. Alternatively, when damage is seen on structural MRI of the basal ganglia, this may be a marker of damage in underlying structures (possible subcortical) where it may not be possible to detect

Table 9.1 Visual deficits associated with cortical and basal ganglia damage.

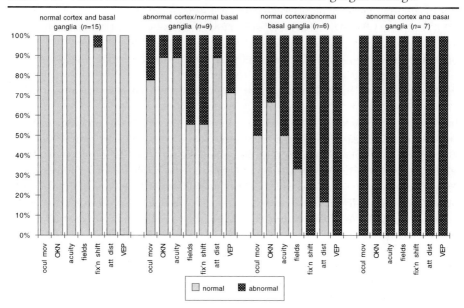

Fig. 9.1 ocul mov = ocular movement; OKN = optokinetic nystagmus; fix'n shift = fixation shifts; att dist = attention at distance; VEP = visual evoked potential.

damage on current paediatric MRI scans. In terms of cerebellar damage, obvious damage to it has been rarely seen on early MRI scans but in certain neurological syndromes there are structural changes seen in the anatomy of the cerebellum. It is not known what this indicates, but it is know that in some syndromes and not others it is linked to marked neurological deficits. In our recent studies, which looked at the brains of two young WS children (see later in this chapter), we suggest that more minor changes in cerebellar structure are not associated with gross neurological problems, although these children show many abnormalities of spatiovisual development and visuomotor development. (Mercuri *et al.* 1997*c*).

In all these studies at least two potentially major problems have been identified. One is the relative sensitivity of our present measures in diagnosing HIE severity, in abnormality as assessed from structural MRI and in our methods for identifying small delays or deficits of early vision. The second problem is that subtle changes in development of the brain at an early stage may not in themselves produce a detectable early visual deficit, but may compromise development of more complex brain circuitry at a later stage. Longitudinal detailed follow-up of these cohorts may enable us with hindsight to tease out further correlations, but a true understanding of causality will require therapeutic interventions whose short- and long-term effects can be tested in randomized controlled trials, if ethically valid protocols can be devised for these.

Overall, our results imply some remarkable plasticity of function, in that children can show visual performance that would be expected to depend on visual cortex, despite very extensive damage to this region. However, there are clear constraints on this plasticity: the loss of one hemisphere is not well compensated for (at least in some critical aspects of visual behaviour), and damage whose visible trace is in the basal ganglia can lead to long-lasting visual deficits, even though these structures had not previously been thought to play a necessary part in all aspects of adult visual function.

9.3.3 Anomalous brain development: the case of Williams syndrome

In the preceding section, conditions were considered where the program of brain development is faced with external disruption; e.g., from a local or general deprivation of oxygen. There are other conditions where the program itself follows an anomalous course: the genetic instructions for building the brain are either imperfect or are prevented from being expressed in the normal way. These conditions also raise questions of plasticity. Can the brain develop towards its normal functional goals by unusual routes? If one aspect of the brain's structure or function is properly expressed, how does it interact with other aspects whose development is absent or abnormal? Do the normally developing parts of the brain expand their development at the expense of the abnormal parts?

These questions have been provoked by the condition known as Williams syndrome (WS). WS is a rare genetically based condition, including a characteristic profile of cognitive development, which is associated with deletion of parts of chromosome 7, the extent of deletion being quite variable across individual cases (Ewert *et al.* 1993; Frangiskakis *et al.* 1996). It has attracted much interest because of the dissociation between the relative sparing of language and face recognition on the one hand, and the severe deficit of spatial cognition on the other (Bellugi *et al.* 1988, 1990). Interestingly, many WS children also appear to develop elaborate linguistic, social, and musical skills; they are often excellent story tellers and competent musicians in playing and remembering music by ear.

Clearly, some systems, involved in the processing of visuospatial information, have been seriously compromised in the brain development of WS children. Other systems dealing with parts of the linguistic domain, notably speech production, appear relatively intact (although often their discourse is different from children with normal development). The nature of brain development and plasticity would be understood much better if it was known whether this reflected independence in development of the two systems, or whether developing linguistic systems have compensated for, or exploited, the anomalies in visuospatial systems. Unfortunately, it is not yet known whether specific brain systems are switched from visual to verbal processing or whether WS brains are only capable of carrying out certain types of processing (useful in linguistic learning but inappropriate in visuospatial learning). Functional brain imaging while carrying out controlled cognitive tasks might reveal some answers to these questions, but its technical demands make it currently impractical for young children, or, probably, for adults with the cognitive level and personality typically found in WS.

The chromosomal abnormality in WS must be expressed at some level in the structure of the brain, but the path through brain structure to cognitive profile is not yet understood. Some differences in the volumetric ratios of different gross brain structures have been found (Jernigan *et al.* 1993). We have found, using structural MRI, that early in development (two young WS children aged 3 years and 2 years 4 months) the cerebellum shows anomalies of size and structure, and that there are also anomalies in certain areas of cerebral white matter (Mercuri *et al.* 1997*c*). The latter may well be related to the connectivity of particular functional mechanisms, but it is not yet known whether we are seeing a persisting abnormality of structure, or a transient developmental phase, perhaps reflecting delay.

9.3.4 Visual and cognitive development in Williams syndrome

Earlier studies of WS have not considered the relation between basic visual mechanisms and spatial cognitive function. They have also tended to concentrate on near-adult cases rather than the developmental course in young children. These were the areas we initially approached in the systematic study of a large group of young UK children with WS between the ages of 12 months and 13 years, which has been carried out since 1993. As this study has developed, it has been possible to focus on more specific questions about the nature of anomalous brain development in WS.

One of the initial aims of the study was to look for any possible visual precursors of visuocognitive deficit in these children, looking at the incidence of basic visual problems such as strabismus, deficits in stereoscopic vision, poor visual acuity, and refractive errors. It was found from an initial questionnaire, returned by 108 families, that along with problems of spatial cognition and action (e.g. difficulty with construction toys such as Lego, and with walking down stairs or over uneven surfaces), there was a high incidence of refractive error and strabismus. This questionnaire was followed up by offering the families fuller detailed assessments in our Unit of all aspects of visual, visuocognitive, and some measures of linguistic, development. Each child spent at least half a day in the Unit with plenty of breaks for social interaction, participating in an extensive set of tests. The full results have been reported elsewhere (Braddick and Atkinson 1995).

From systematic follow-up assessment of these children it was found that approximately half failed a standard orthoptic examination, failed the standard stereo tests (TNO and Lang), showed marked refractive errors for their age and acuity falling below age norms, even when these norms were in terms of their age equivalence on verbal IQ, rather than their chronological age. Interestingly, most of their refractive errors were hyperopic rather than myopic, supporting the idea that such neurologically compromised groups may be slow emmetropizers (as most of the group were already over 6 years of age, by which age emmetropization is thought to be complete in normal populations).

A large group of these children was tested on a number of visuospatial tasks, some taken from our own assessment battery and some from standard paediatric tests. Examples in Fig. 9.7 of the calculated age equivalents on two of these spatial tests serves to show their difficulties within the spatial domain. There is also a wide range of deficits across the group, with some children showing much larger deficits than others.

Results on the block construction tests, and on the object-assembly subtest of the

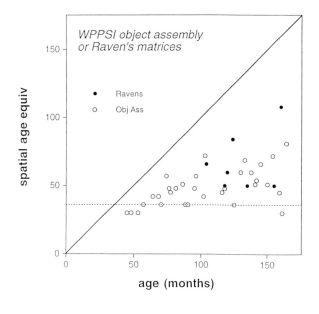

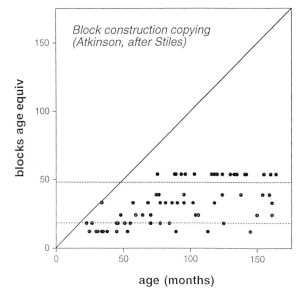

Fig. 9.7 Calculated developmental age equivalents for WS children (aged 2–13 years) on the ABCDEFV block copying task and other standard spatial tasks (WPPSI object assembly and Raven's Matrices Test). Each point represents the result for one child. On the block construction task a group of the WS children were able to copy the most complex construction in the battery and so were at ceiling on this task. Their results are shown as single points above the 50- month dotted line. Other WS children do not develop beyond the normal 4 year old level, no matter what their chronological age. WPPSI = Wechsler Preschool and Primary Scale of Intelligence.

Wechsler Preschool and Primary Scale of Intelligence (WPPSI) test, both show (in Fig. 9.7) that in many cases WS children do not develop beyond that of a normal 4 year old. Several neuroscientific hypotheses are being considered, concerning the differences in brain development, which might underlie the characteristic WS performance, and these are briefly discussed below.

9.3.4.1 *Hypothesis 1: visual and spatial deficits are strongly linked*

Could the problems of acuity, refraction, and binocularity that have been seen, be precursors of the spatial difficulties in WS—either part of the causal chain or reflecting a common mechanism? This might be an attractively simple hypothesis.

From comparisons to date, when we look at whether there is a significant correlation between the extent of the spatial deficit and presence of sensory visual deficits (such as lack of stereopsis, strabismus, poor acuity) in individual WS children, no evidence of a clear relationship is found. For example, in Fig. 9.8 deficits in stereo vision do not seem to be associated with the level of performance on tests of spatial construction and cognition. Individual WS children, showing severe delays in spatial development may show no sensory visual deficits and WS children with marked sensory visual deficits may show milder deficits on spatial tasks than those without sensory deficits.

9.3.4.2 *Hypothesis 2: Dorsal stream deficit*

The evidence that face recognition is spared whereas spatial problems are widespread in WS suggests a plausible link between WS deficits and the functioning of the

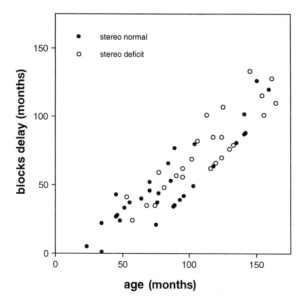

Fig. 9.8 Comparison of WS children with and without stereoscopic deficits in the extent of their delays (in age equivalence) on the block construction task.

dorsal cortical stream. This pathway, referred to in a number of preceding chapters, has been supposed to encode, beyond the primary visual cortex, information about spatial relationships (Mishkin *et al.* 1983) and the visual control of action (Glickstein and May 1982; Milner and Goodale 1995). In contrast, face recognition is a prime example of the function of the ventral stream leading to the temporal lobe. We have gained support for the idea of a dorsal deficit in WS, by finding a specific deficit in many WS children in their performance on a task requiring detection of global motion, and in a second task of visuomanual control.

9.3.4.2.1 Motion and form coherence

Chapter 3 pointed out that cortical area V5 (MT) is a key structure in the dorsal stream, and contains neurons with large, directionally selective receptive fields which are highly sensitive to coherent global motion in the presence of noise (Britten *et al.* 1992). Motion coherence thresholds are severely impaired by lesions of V5 in macaques (Newsome and Paré 1988) and humans (Baker *et al.* 1991). Thus, motion coherence thresholds provide a test of dorsal stream function. To ensure that any deficit in WS was not simply a general problem with psychophysical judgements on global stimuli, motion coherence thresholds were tested alongside a new task designed to place comparable demands on the ventral stream (Atkinson *et al.* 1997). The stimuli used for these measurements have already been illustrated in Chapter 7 (Fig. 7.5). In the 'dorsal stream' task, subjects had to locate a strip of random dots, oscillating in opposite phase to those in the surround, as the percentage of dots in purely random motion was progressively increased. (This is a display that has also been successfully used with infants: Wattam-Bell 1994.) In the 'ventral stream' task, subjects had to locate a region in which short line segments were oriented tangentially to concentric circles, with the rest of the display containing randomly oriented line segments; the percentage of randomly oriented segments within the circle region was progressively increased This is designed to test the processing of static form by ventral areas; in particular, neurons responding to concentric arrangements have been reported in V4 (Galant *et al.* 1993).

Figure 9.9 shows the coherence thresholds for both motion and static form of our WS children, compared with the mean coherence thresholds for a large group of normal controls aged between 4 years and 8 years. The WS children show somewhat higher values than many of the normal children on motion coherence, but many have form coherence thresholds within the normal range. For some of the WS children their relative performance on motion and form coherence is similar to that of a normal 4–5 year old, with much better performance on the form coherence task than the motion. It is as though development for this type of motion processing has stopped or slowed down at the 4-year-old level and cannot progress and improve.

9.3.4.2.2 The letter box task—matching orientation and posting

It has been proposed that the dorsal stream is not just generally concerned with locations and relationships in space, but specifically processes this information to guide

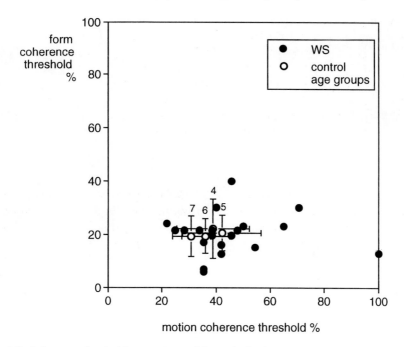

Fig. 9.9 Coherence thresholds—motion and form, for both WS children and normal controls.

actions, in particular those of the hand. One piece of evidence comes for a patient, believed to have damage in ventral stream structures, who can fluently insert a card into a slot of variable orientation, but completely fails to match visually the seen orientation of the same slot (Milner and Goodale 1995).

This test was adapted for children to look at whether the reverse dissociation could be seen in WS children on this task (Atkinson *et al.* 1997). The results of these tests are shown in Fig. 9.10, together with a picture of a child posting the letter in an adapted post-box. Most of the WS children really enjoyed posting the letters, although many of them did not plan the posting action well and were very inaccurate (as seen in Fig. 9.10).

Some WS children had more difficulty in understanding the matching-without-posting task, but nevertheless were more accurate on it than in the posting part of the task. On posting, normal 4 year olds show 7–15° errors with mean errors of 4–10° for older children and adults. Only two of the WS children performed within this range, and five WS children had very large errors with the orientation of the letter, which was almost uncorrelated with the angle of the slot. The letter was often posted in these cases by trial and error, rather than by any evident attempt to match orientation visually. For the two WS children who achieved normal levels of accuracy in posting, it was interesting to see that they sometimes showed indications of compensatory strategies. Rather than making a rapid automatic posting action, they first looked at the slot, then slowly lifted the letter and advanced it towards the letter box.

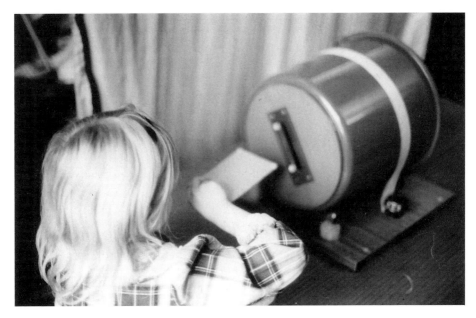

Fig. 9.10(a)

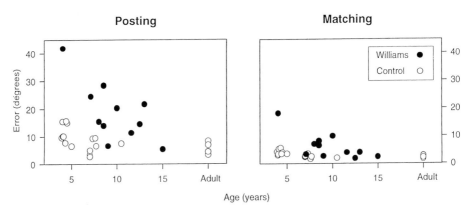

Fig. 9.10(b)

Fig. 9.10 (a) child inaccurately posting the letter. (b) Posting and matching results for WS children and controls. For posting, the mean angle of error for each child when the letter edge was 2 cm away from the slot, calculated from the Elite records of the hand trajectory, is plotted. For matching the mean angle of error set by the child on the mannequin's letter, is plotted.

As their hand and arm moved, they checked the letter position and the orientation of the slot. This did not look like an 'automatic' action, but rather a series of small actions which were continually checked visually.

There are, therefore, good indications of a dorsal stream deficit in at least some of the WS children assessed on both the post-box task and the motion coherence measures. Such a deficit would help to explain the specific difficulties found in WS for tasks such as block construction, object assembly, and drawing; it might also contribute to their reported difficulties in locomotion over physically or visually uneven surfaces (Withers 1996). However, the degree of variation found in the group, and other aspects of their pattern of deficit, make it unlikely that a dorsal stream deficit is the only neural basis for cognitive and performance anomalies in WS.

9.3.4.3 Hypothesis 3: Frontal deficits

One common characteristic of WS children is that they seem to have very limited attention spans and are easily distracted by the surrounding environment; for example, by sounds outside the testing room. However, on occasions they show extreme persistence to repeat certain acts over and over again in a stereotypic fashion (e.g. listening to the same tune over and over again on a musical box, repeating the same question over and over again even if the question is always answered). Both of these types of behaviour are reported for adult patients with frontal cortical damage.

There is some evidence that many WS children show frontal deficits, which may be shown up either in the verbal domain or in the visuospatial domain. Two tasks that we have used both involve suppressing or inhibiting a familiar, overlearned, response while executing a newly learnt association. One task is an adaptation of the Stroop test, called the day–night test, which we were introduced to by Adele Diamond (see Diamond *et al.* 1997; Adele Diamond has used the test for looking at frontal problems in children with phenylketonuria). The child has to say 'day' to a picture depicting the night sky, and 'night' to a picture of the sun. This is the reverse of the nomally associated response. Another frontal task we have used is an adaptation of our own fixation shift display, for a task which is called *counterpointing*. It is similar to the antisaccade tasks that have been used to test frontal function in adults. In the pointing/counterpointing task the child has to point as rapidly as possible when the target appears, either on the same side of the screen as the target ('pointing'), i.e. pointing to the target, or to the opposite side of the screen to the target ('counter pointing'), i.e. away from the target (Fig. 9.11 (b)). After one or two practice trials, normal children over the age of 4 years can perform both these tasks rapidly and automatically. The mean latencies for the two responses are much the same when the task is automated. WS children with verbal IQ scores 4 years or above were tested on the pointing/counterpointing tasks and the results are shown in Fig. 9.11 (a).

On the day–night test the WS children can be divided into two groups: there are those who perform like normal children over the age of 7 years and can inhibit the familiar association between the word and picture, and there are those who can perform the control task of paired association learning but cannot carry out the Stroop task—they cannot inhibit their familiar responses in the day–night task. They revert to saying 'day' to the picture of the sun, and 'night' to the picture of the moon.

On the pointing/counterpointing task we have compared each child's mean latency for pointing to the correct side, and counterpointing to the opposite side to the target. Even the older WS children often show much longer delays in counterpointing than do young normal children. Very few of the WS children ever seemed to be able to achieve an automatic counterpoint: even when they could successfully do the task and did not revert to pointing to the target as it appeared, they often had to verbally cue themselves by saying 'opposite side' as they made the response. This again would imply that they are using a somewhat different strategy to the normal controls. It is as though they have to inhibit the familiar response afresh on each trial and cannot easily change their strategy to inhibit the familiar response. On both the day–night task and the pointing–counterpointing task many of the WS children, over the verbal mental age of 4 years, would appear to show deficits similar to frontal adult patients. One of our current projects is to compare different frontal marker tasks in these children to discover whether it is a generalized frontal deficit, or a specific deficit of development in particular parietofrontal circuits.

9.3.4.4 Right and left hemisphere deficits

There is considerable evidence that the right hemisphere has a particular role in the processing and representation of spatial representations. In development, this has

Fig. 9.11(a)

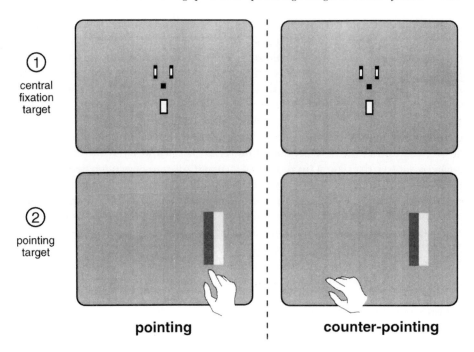

Fig. 9.11 (a) Pointing compared with counterpointing mean latencies for WS children and normal controls (over 4 years of age). Some of the WS children have long counterpointing latencies. Some WS children also make errors in that they point rather than counterpoint. (b) Schematic representation of the pointing and counterpointing task.

been illustrated by Joan Stiles' work showing that the right hemisphere focal lesions have a greater effect than left on children's performance in block constructions (Stiles-Davis *et al*. 1985; Stiles and Nass 1991). Language, on the other hand, is well known to be dominated by left hemisphere processing.

As WS children are often linguistically fluent, but show extreme difficulty with block construction, it is tempting to suggest that their problems are predominantly associated with the right hemisphere, perhaps particularly with the right parietal lobe. In adult stroke patients, neglect of the left side of space is a common feature of right-sided lesions. Therefore, 'neglect-like' behaviour might be expected under certain circumstances in WS. However, the fixation shift task (described in Chapter 8) in older WS children showed no evidence of a unilateral deficit of left space (right hemisphere), even in the 'competition condition', which might be closer to the conditions of neglect testing than the non-competition condition. While it might be of interest to test WS with closer analogues to neuropsychological tests of neglect (e.g. cancellation tasks), there is not yet any evidence known that specifically offers strong support for the idea of interhemispheric differences in WS.

Figure 9.12 depicts a speculative, but hopefully plausible, model of how brain development in WS might reflect a plastic system that starts off on an anomalous developmental course. As suggested earlier, normally development of both cortical streams takes off after birth, with a possible small general delay in the first postnatal months in WS and then the normal lead for ventral over dorsal stream development. In normal development a surge in dorsal stream development occurs late in the first and in the second year of life, but this surge may be further delayed in WS and the system may not be quite as plastic as in normal development. In normal 1–3 year olds, language processing and the control of skilled, spatially directed actions are developing rapidly in parallel. WS children generally show delays both in the onset of language and in the development of motor actions. However, if the delay for language is shorter than for actions, the balance and relative developmental timing of these two domains is upset and desynchronized. Language systems become effectively coupled to emotional and social activities (but much less so to dorsal-stream-based spatial and action representations). This is followed by language systems expanding their connectivity at the expense of the dorsal stream systems, which never recover from their initial delay and reduced plasticity.

It may also be supposed that an important part of frontal functioning is initially built, in normal development, for the control, selection, and inhibition of signals that drive eye and hand movements. In WS there is a developmental deficit in the dorsal-stream parietal systems that provide these signals, leading to a knock-on effect in frontal control functions. This does not, however, provide a clear account of the day/night Stroop effect deficit, as it does not propose a reason for delay in the linkage between language and frontal systems. One possibility is a mismatch in timing between the exuberance of speech production at 3–4 years in WS and the normal course of frontal development. The inhibition of a prepotent speech response in the Stroop situation requires appropriate synchrony between frontal control systems and articulatory mechanisms. This is an even more speculative idea, but it would be interesting to see if it could be expressed in neural network models which had to

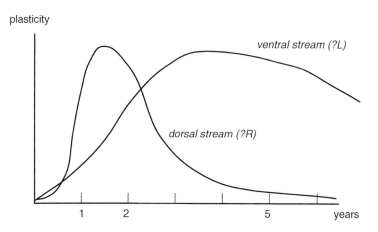

Fig. 9.12 Speculative model of the plasticity of different cortical streams within brain development in WS child.

develop the relative timing of initially independent temporal pattern generators. I leave readers with this extremely speculative scheme and hope that you will provide further experimental evidence to either confirm or negate the more speculative parts of it.

9.4 OVERVIEW

Plasticity in development is one of the most pervasive questions in psychology, neuroscience, and biology generally. Our experience in studying vision in a wide variety of clinical paediatric conditions makes us also aware of its human and practical implications. The hopes of every parent whose child has suffered a perinatal brain insult, or early cataract or squint, depend on the belief in plasticity of brain systems.

In the face of this, I am very conscious of the somewhat fragmentary nature of our knowledge. Ten years ago, elegant experiments on cats and primates had demonstrated the plasticity of binocular cortical organization. These have provided some guidance on what can be expected from surgery and occlusion therapies for unilateral and bilateral deprivation, e.g. from dense cataract. However, it is not understood how far the effects known in V1 underlie ordinary amblyopia associated with squint or refractive error. Nor do we really understand the fragility of binocularity when it is restored by strabismus surgery, perhaps because we do not really understand the relationships between accommodation, refractive error, convergence and disparity processing which led to the squint in the first place.

The visual input to the cortex is organized in a relatively simple and ordered way, to create the topographic cortical layout and its specific receptive field types. If this organization is the result of an input-dependent plastic system rather than a rigid program, it seems certain that at least as much plasticity must be required to build up the richer and more flexible systems that represent objects and their spatial relations, and determine the overall flow of information and control within the brain. However, very little is known about how the child's experience, transmitted through the earlier stages of visual processing, determines organization at these levels.

We see children who recover from apparently massive cortical damage at birth. These cases lead us to believe that the brain can exploit its own plasticity as a self-organizing system, and give us hope that we may someday be able to provide inputs that guide this plasticity more effectively. At the same time, other small lesions seem to have a much more permanently damaging effect. When these differences have been understood, it may be possible to identify the role of certain brain systems in guiding the flexible development of the rest. In the meantime, research continues on the cellular and molecular basis for neuronal survival and recovery. It is hoped that it will be possible to link this with an understanding of development at functional and systems levels.

If we compare across the various examples of anomalous development considered in this chapter, a common theme is the vulnerability of the functioning of the dorsal stream compared with the ventral stream—vulnerability of binocular interactions, motion coherence, and visuomotor actions. This vulnerability has also been seen in some subgroups of visual dyslexics (for example, in raised motion coherence thresholds) and recently it was found in hemiplegic children, who show raised motion coherence thresholds compared with form coherence thresholds (Atkinson *et al.* 1999). However, vulnerability is not restricted to the dorsal stream. Many aspects of amblyopia would seem to involve processing in both the dorsal and ventral streams and cortical orientation processing (when using the VEP measure to gauge onset of cortical processing) does seem to indicate that vulnerability of both dorsal and ventral streams, and the interactions between them, underlies abnormal development in many paediatric patients.

10   Concluding remarks

10.1   WHAT IS OUR CURRENT MODEL OF VISUAL BRAIN DEVELOPMENT?

Knowledge of the infant visual brain has grown in 25 years from almost nothing to a rich, complex, but sometimes puzzling set of findings. Some of the puzzles require more patient and ingenious experimentation of the kind that has brought us so far; some await a better understanding of the mature visual brain; and some depend on advances in the tricky techniques that can bring together scientific precision with the uncertainties and fleeting opportunities of working with babies.

The principal theme of this book has been the development of cortical function. In many of our early studies, this was a two-pronged attack to analyse, first, specialized attribute detectors and, secondly, how they were selected in early selective attentional processing. We focused our findings on postnatal development of specialized cortical detectors sensitive to properties that are known to be processed in primary visual cortex, area V1. These were three spatial attributes: orientation (necessary for shape analysis); directional movement (for segmenting objects and ordering them in depth, analysing their trajectories, and identifying biologically significant events); and binocular correlation and disparity (for analysing 3-D shape, surface, and distance).

These detector properties did not appear to develop all together, and the differences may be analysed in terms of the distinction between the magnocellular and parvocellular pathways to and through visual cortex. The later developing functions (motion and disparity analysis) have both been identified primarily with the magnocellular pathway. Orientation sensitivity appears earlier after birth. Although our own studies have not considered colour sensitivity, data from other laboratories suggested that responses to isoluminant colour displays could also be seen in the first 2 months. Orientation (form) and colour are the properties whose analysis is generally identified with the parvocellular pathway. Thus, at least in terms of functional properties, the parvo system appears to be somewhat advanced on the magno system in the months after birth.

These two streams of visual processing continue, of course, beyond the primary detectors found in V1. Indeed, we do not yet know how far the factors that limit infants' developing sensitivities to orientation, motion, and disparity actually lie in the V1 detectors and how far in subsequent processing. Information about these attributes is relayed through extrastriate visual areas, in the ventral and dorsal streams respectively. A major challenge for the future is to develop behavioural and visual evoked potential methods that can distinguish clearly between the successive stages of processing in each of these streams. This task will be helped by functional imaging studies, where we are starting to isolate the processing which occurs in each of the many human visual areas, and establish more firmly the homologies between human visual brain and structures which have been investigated in other primates.

The division between dorsal and ventral streams is a major aspect of brain organization, but it cannot be absolute. Abilities such as reaching for a particular identified object, or using patterns of motion to recognize a human being, imply that information analysed in one stream can be fed into another. The story of infant visual development must, therefore, include the integration of these streams as well as the development and refinement of function within each stream. This idea has been hinted at in previous developmental studies. For example, Bower (1974) suggested that infants up to about 5 months of age identified an object either in its static form or when moving along a trajectory—a static and moving object were treated as two distinct objects by very young infants, as though the analysis of dynamic and static input information was initially uncoordinated and then integrated.

Furthermore, the idea of analysis proceeding from 'lower' to higher' levels, either within or between streams, is at best an incomplete guide to visual brain function. Advances in neurobiology in recent years have made our views of visual cortical function considerably richer and more complex. It has become clear that there is a wealth of 'descending' as well as 'ascending' pathways between cortical visual areas, and also multiple pathways (in both directions) between cortical and subcortical visual structures. Some important aspects of development, including the control of attention, optokinetic responses, and second-order processing are all likely to involve one or both of these kinds of pathway.

Our studies of abnormal development suggest that there is differential vulnerability for different parts of this system. Binocular interaction seems to be particularly delicate and easily disrupted, so strabismus and loss of binocularity is a common feature of children with perinatal brain insults, and of developmental disorders including Williams' syndrome, as well as being associated with abnormal relationships between refraction, accommodation, and vergence. This might be attributed to the stringent requirements of precise binocular co-ordination, rather than the dorsal-stream nature of disparity processing as such. However, other developmental disorders of vision seem to be much more associated with the dorsal rather than the ventral stream. The dorsal motion coherence test was found to show more problems than the ventral form coherence test in Williams syndrome children, but this is probably not highly specific to this syndrome; hemiplegic children also show a proportionately greater deficit in motion than form coherence, and developmental dyslexics have also been shown to have higher motion coherence thresholds. Attentional deficits also are a common feature of neurological problems and go hand in hand with the binocular and motion problems. On the other hand, cortical problems that might be specifically associated with the ventral stream, such as prosopagnosia (deficit in face recognition) and central colour deficits, are very rare in children. Hopefully, precise analysis of early structural brain imaging, and identifying varying degrees of dorsal–ventral imbalance in different children, may help to throw light on the reasons for this apparent differential vulnerability. Our conclusions, at present, concerning development of the dorsal and ventral stream, would seem to be that something about the early integration and processing of the dorsal stream makes it very vulnerable to disruption, and this is not true of ventral stream processing.

One system of cortical and subcortical structures, which remains mysterious but clearly important, is the basal ganglia. Pathways looping from the cortex through the basal ganglia to the thalamus and back to the cortex have been mapped out, but their main role has been considered to be in the selection and execution of motor, including oculomotor, programs. It can be seen from Chapter 9 that apparently quite small lesions in the basal ganglia can have rather severe effects on visual development, which go beyond problems that have an obvious oculomotor involvement. Do these loops play a part in the setting up of cortical visual processing, even if they have no evident role in this processing in the adult? Fuller and more detailed comparisons of infant and adult patients may provide the way forward here.

A warning on the interpretation of these anatomical data comes from a different structure—the cerebellum. In severe perinatal brain damage, post-mortem examination often shows severe damage to the cerebellum. And yet, it is rather rare to identify this damage on magnetic resonance imaging. The implication is that imaging may give us a rather partial view of the state of the brain: perhaps the damage we can see, in basal ganglia or elsewhere, is just a token of wider invisible damage. As the technologies of imaging become more refined and diverse, we may get a very different picture.

10.2 GIVEN OUR CURRENT MODEL, WHAT IS VISION REALLY LIKE FOR YOUNG INFANTS?

Many loose ends and unfinished questions will have been apparent throughout this book, as well as in this closing overview. I have not attempted to gloss over the cracks but left them wide open for the future. The most obvious, and yet the most difficult question is: *what is the visual world of the infant really like?* For example, before 8 weeks the infant shows no sign of being able to make motion-based discriminations. Yet, a dynamic stimulus is attention-getting—it represents some kind of attractive activity. Even its specific direction of movement is available to oculomotor mechanisms and reflected in some presumably cortical signals. What is it like to be alerted by motion, to respond to it, and yet in most respects apparently not to see it as having a direction? What happens when your mother walks by?

Similarly, it seems likely that putting together object properties is a slow and uncertain process in early infancy. Does this mean that objects are fragmented for infants, a set of attributes which are present in perception but somehow do not cohere in space and time? Or are they represented by only the simplest and most prominent features or affordances, for example, in a face with only those features which undergo minimal transformation with movement of the head? Is this the same as saying that the particular stage of development of the infant's cortical selective attentional mechanisms will decide which feature is most salient?

10.3 THE ROLE OF CONSCIOUSNESS AND CONTROL

Asking these questions in such a form perhaps may be mistaken, if they imply that infants and young children have a unified visual consciousness. The neural underpinnings of conscious experience in adults are currently an issue for active debate by many eminent neuroscientists, such as Francis Crick, Semir Zeki, Larry Weiskrantz, and Alan Cowey. Some argue that consciousness is associated with particular forms of activity—such as highly temporally coherent activity—which may appear very widely across the brain. Such activity may be evoked or modulated by generalized attentional circuits, but they are not unique to particular structures in the brain and may not even necessarily be unified. Others argue that the activity of certain brain areas intrinsically do not reach consciousness directly, and awareness is a property of certain distinct sites in the brain. Neither approach leads to direct hypotheses about visual consciousness in infants, but they would point to very different ways to look for evidence in the infant brain.

My own view is that the changes we see in alertness and visual behaviour in the first 3–4 months look like the emergence of an active, self-controlled, information-seeking perceiver. If we can ever accept that consciousness is present in a creature who cannot describe it, we would have to accept it in an infant of this age. Given the evidence that the changes reflect cortical functioning, I would propose that consciousness is a function of the cortical areas that are primarily involved in early selective attention. However, it could also be argued that this early consciousness is qualitatively different from the consciousness that can be shared with other individuals. At 3 or 4 years, children can start to show evidence of reflections on their own mental processes—what psychologists call *metacognition*—and communicate their understanding that another individual has an inner life that includes thoughts, wishes, and beliefs like their own—*theory of mind*.

This more advanced, and more unambiguous stage of consciousness involves the operation of executive processes that can monitor, modulate, and control the flow of other cognitive processes. There is much evidence that such processes depend on the circuitry of the frontal lobes. However, current thinking about executive function is that it is not unitary but can be fractionated (Shallice and Burgess 1996). The nature of such fractionation must be considered when tests for frontal control processes are looked at, an area we have begun research on in the Visual Development Unit, as input to such control represents one of the goals of visual information processing.

Different tests are appropriate for different ages. At 1 year of age, delay in the Piagetian search task known as 'A-not-B' provides a means to test the child's ability to inhibit a prepotent response, and has been related by Adele Diamond and colleagues (1997) with the function of frontal area 46. At later ages other tests provide more sensitive indicators of response inhibition, such as the Day-Night Stroop test and the counterpointing test, which have been described in the context of Williams syndrome in Chapter 9. Does the progression between these tasks simply represent a quantitative increase in the complexity of task which can be communicated to the child, or does it represent a transition between different types of control process, perhaps associated with qualitative changes in the kind of conscious monitoring which the child can bring to the processing of the input? We do not know, but it is clear that any progress in understanding consciousness in relation to vision, in children or adults, cannot stop with the visual mechanisms at the back of the brain but must consider how these communicate with control mechanisms at the front.

10.4 HOW MUCH PLASTICITY AND VARIATION IS THERE IN DEVELOPMENT?

In attempting to formulate a model of development of the visual brain, the milestones which define a single, normal developmental route have been emphasized. Certainly, there are striking similarities across children in the sequence and timing in which functions and mechanisms emerge. However, Chapter 9 discussed the broad issue of plasticity. It is clear the development is not the unfolding of a fixed plan, but can follow routes that are dependent on the individual's experience. Further, there are wide individual differences in the behavioural patterns, emotional moods, and social styles of different infants, and in the same infant over time. What is the balance between individuality and conformity to a developmental plan in the developing brain, and how is it maintained to achieve the end-point goals of development?

Is plasticity itself a matter of individual difference, and if so what are the limiting factors that control it? Some of us can learn a new language at 70 years and some of us can't. Does this kind of difference reflect a variation in underlying plasticity, or does it reflect the kind of cognitive structures that have been developed in an early, but limited, plastic period?

In earlier chapters all these issues of nature–nurture interactions have been touched upon, but it seems that at present we can only predict an individual's course of visual development in the rather broad terms of 'normal' and 'abnormal'; and the range of abnormality (as discussed in Chapter 9) is very wide.

10.5 WHAT IS VISUAL DISABILITY?

When plasticity is inadequate to maintain the developmental course in the face of damage, visual disability may result. However, this term raises its own questions, especially when used in the developing child. Disability implies an impact on the quality of the child's life. Children at different ages have different needs, both for their immediate life and to provide the foundations for future development. They also have different cognitive abilities at different ages. The evaluation of vision problems, therefore requires an understanding of both the child's level of cognitive ability and the child's changing needs (including both spatial skills and linguistic communication level), as well as an appreciation of the dynamic process by which the child builds new skills upon earlier achievements.

As can be seen in Chapter 9 the course of development can be disturbed by factors operating at many different levels and different stages of development. Often, in individual cases, it is not known where the prime area of the problem lies or how effective remediation would be provided. Given the difficulties of defining the causes of abnormal development, and its effects in terms of disability, I am sure of one thing. It will take considerable co-operation and humility between different professional groups, each trained and possessing different skills, if we are to pin-point disability and make any sense of it.

If we are to gain any real insights into successful treatments, it will require well controlled randomized trials which are humane, ethical, and practical within existing health management systems. It will often be necessary to admit that professional 'clinical wisdom' does not provide adequate answers. Practically, however, professionals, while remaining aware of the limitations of scientific and clinical knowledge, have to give advice to parents and carers which is supportive and useful. In giving this advice we have to understand the variations between families in their robustness and tolerance of uncertainty. We need education in cultural, social and ethical issues, to be able to communicate our findings so that they can be understood by those we are attempting to help and we need to learn how to communicate with the public and enter the wider societal debate. At the same time, we need to consider paediatric visual problems in the light of all paediatric health problems. There are always going to be limited resources and we must liaise with health professionals, engaged in public health issues involving cost-effectiveness and cost-benefit analyses, if we are to progress not only our understanding of visual disability but to provide useful expertise to those caring for children with problems. Most of all we must be willing to learn from others.

10.6 HOW CAN WE WORK ACROSS MULTIPLE LEVELS OF ANALYSIS?

Both normal and abnormal visual development have been addressed through many different techniques, working across different levels of analysis. We have touched on findings and ideas from neuroscience, including electrophysiology, anatomy, and functional imaging, from pharmacology and analyses at the cellular and molecular levels, from behavioural experiments and observations, from psychological models and theories, and from the approach of the neurological or ophthalmological clinician. The language and concepts from these different approaches may be hard to bring together, but none of them is going to give us an adequate understanding on its own and each contributes pieces to the jigsaw puzzle. We must learn to be patient and tolerant in trying to grasp the questions asked in each others' approaches, and support each others' efforts. Always remember that the strongest force in the advancement of science is serendipity—which comes from openness to new ideas—combined with careful hard work. You never know where the next breakthrough is coming from but it helps to remain optimistic!

References

Adams, R. J., Maurer, D., and Cashin, H. A. (1990). The influence of stimulus size on newborns' discrimination of chromatic from achromatic stimuli. *Vision Research*, **30**, 2023–2030.

Adelson, E. H. and Bergen, J. R. (1985). Spatiotemporal energy models for the perception of motion. *Journal of the Optical Society of America*, **A2**, 284–299.

Allen, D., Banks, M. S., and Schefrin, B. (1988). Chromatic discrimination in human infants, a re-examination. *Investigative Ophthalmology and Visual Science (Suppl.)* **29**, 25.

Allen, D., Banks, M. S., Norcia, A. M., and Shannon, L. (1993). Does chromatic sensitivity develop more slowly than luminance sensitivity? *Vision Research*, **33**, 2553–2562.

Allport, A. (1989). Visual attention. In M. I. Posner (Ed.), *Foundations of cognitive science*, pp. 631–682. Cambridge, MA: MIT Press.

Anker, S., Atkinson, J., and MacIntyre, A. M. (1989). The use of the Cambridge Crowding Cards in preschool vision screening programmes, ophthalmic clinics and assessment of children with multiple disabilities. *Ophthalmic and Physiological Optics*, **9**, 470.

Anker, S., Atkinson, J., Braddick, O., Ehrlich, D., Wade, J., and Weeks, F. (1995). Screening for strabismus and refractive errors in the Cambridge Health District, a comparison between cycloplegic and non-cycloplegic techniques: First results. *Strabismus*, **3**, 191.

Anstis, S. M. and Cavanagh, P. (1983). A minimum motion technique for judging equiluminance. In J. D. Mollon and L. T. Sharp (Eds), *Color vision: physiology and psychophysics*. London: Academic Press.

Apkarian, P. (1996). Chiasmal crossing defects in disorders of binocular vision. *Eye*, **10**, 222–231.

Appelle, S. (1972). Perception and discrimination as a function of stimulus orientation: the 'oblique effect' in man and animals. *Psychological Bulletin*, **78**, 266–278.

Arbib, M. A. (1985). Schemas for the temporal organization of behaviour. *Human Neurobiology*, **4**, 63–72.

Archer, S. M. (1993). Detection and treatment of congenital esotropia. In K. Simons (Ed.), *Early visual development: normal and abnormal*, pp. 349–363. New York: Oxford University Press

Aslin, R. N. (1981). Development of smooth pursuit in human infants. In D. F. Fisher, R. A. Monty, and J. W. Senders (Eds), *Eye movements: cognition and visual perception*, pp. 31–52. Hillsdale, NJ: Lawrence Erlbaum Associates.

Aslin, R. N. (1993). Infant accommodation and convergence. In K. Simons (Ed.), *Early visual development: normal and abnormal*, pp. 30–38. New York: Oxford University Press.

Aslin R. N. and Jackson, R. W. (1979). Accommodative-convergence in young infants. *Canadian Journal of Psychology*, **33**, 1671–1678.

Aslin, R. N. and Salapatek, P. (1975). Saccadic localization of targets by the very young human infant. *Perception and Psychophysics*, **17**, 293–302.

Aslin, R. N., Shea, S. L., and Metz, H. S. (1990). Use of the Canon R-1 autorefractor to measure refractive errors and accommodative responses in human infants. *Clinical Vision Science*, **5**, 61–70.

Atkinson, J. (1984). Human visual development over the first six months of life. A review and a hypothesis. *Human Neurobiology*, **3**, 61–74.

Atkinson, J. (1979). Development of optokinetic nystagmus in the human infant and monkey infant: an analogue to development in kittens. In R. D. Freeman (Ed.), *Developmental neurobiology of vision*, pp. 277–288. NATO Advanced Study Institute Series. New York: Plenum Press.

Atkinson, J. (1989). New tests of vision screening and assessment in infants and young children. In J. H. French, S. Harel, and P. Casaer (Eds), *Child neurology and developmental disabilities* (pp. 219–227). Baltimore: Paul H Brookes Publishing Co.

Atkinson, J. (1991). Review of human visual development: crowding and dyslexia. In J. F. Stein (Ed.), *Vision and visual dyslexia*. Vol. 13, *Vision and visual dysfunction* (pp. 44–57). London: MacMillan Press.

Atkinson, J. (1992). Early visual development: differential functioning of parvocellular and magnocellular pathways. *Eye*, **6**, 129–135.

Atkinson, J. (1993). Infant vision screening: prediction and prevention of strabismus and amblyopia from refractive screening in the Cambridge photorefraction programme. In K. Simons (Ed.), *Early visual development: normal and abnormal* (pp. 335–348). New York: Oxford University Press.

Atkinson, J. (1996). Issues in infant vision screening and assessment. In F. Vital-Durand, O. Braddick, and J. Atkinson (Eds), *Infant Vision*, pp. 135–152. Oxford University Press.

Atkinson, J. and Braddick, O. J. (1976). Stereoscopic discrimination in infants. *Perception*, **5**, 29–38.

Atkinson, J. and Braddick, O. J. (1981*a*). Acuity, contrast sensitivity and accommodation in infancy. In R. N. Aslin, J. R. Alberts, and M. R. Petersen (Eds), *The development of perception* Vol. 2 (pp. 245–278). New York: Academic Press.

Atkinson, J. and Braddick, O. J. (1981*b*). Development of optokinetic nystagmus in infants: an indicator of cortical binocularity? In D. F. Fisher, R. A. Monty, and J. W. Senders (Eds), *Eye movements: cognition and visual perception*, pp. 53–66. Hillsdale, NJ: Lawrence Erlbaum Associates.

Atkinson, J. and Braddick, O. J. (1985). Early development of the control of visual attention, *Perception*, **14**, A25.

Atkinson, J. and Braddick, O. J. (1986). Population vision screening and individual visual assessment. *Documenta Ophthalmologica Proceedings Series*, **45**, 376–391.

Atkinson, J. and Braddick, O. (1989). Newborn contrast sensitivity measures: do VEP, OKN and FPL reveal differential development of cortical and subcortical streams? *Investigative Ophthalmology and Visual Science (Suppl.)*, **30**, 311.

Atkinson, J. and Braddick, O. J. (1993). Visual segmentation of oriented textures by infants. *Behavioural Brain Research*, 49, 123–131.

Atkinson, J. and Braddick, O. (1998). Research methods in infant vision. In J. G. Robson and R. H. S. Carpenter (Eds), *Vision research: a practical approach*, pp. 161–186. Oxford University Press.

Atkinson, J. and French, J. (1983). Reaching for rattles: a preliminary study of contrast sensitivity in 7–10 month old infants. *Perception,* 12, A20.

Atkinson, J. and Hood, B. (1997). Development of visual attention. In J. A. Burack and J. T. Enns (Eds), *Attention, Development, and Psychopathology*, pp. 31–54: New York. The Guildford Press.

Atkinson, J. and Van Hof-van Duin, J. (1993). Assessment of normal and abnormal vision during the first years of life. In A. Fielder and M. Bax (Eds), *Management of visual handicap in childhood*, pp. 9–29. London: Mac Keith Press.

Atkinson, J., Braddick, O. J., and Braddick, F. (1974). Acuity and contrast sensitivity of infant vision. *Nature*, 247, 403–404.

Atkinson, J., Braddick O. J., and French, J. (1979). Contrast sensitivity of the human neonate measured by the visual evoked potential. *Investigative Ophthalmology and Visual Science*, 18, 210–213.

Atkinson, J., Braddick, O. J., and French, J. (1980). Infant astigmatism: Its disappearance with age. *Vision Research*, 20, 891–893.

Atkinson, J., Braddick, O. J., and Pimm-Smith, E. (1982). 'Preferential looking' for monocular and binocular acuity testing of infants. *British Journal of Ophthalmology*, 66, 264–268.

Atkinson, J., Pimm-Smith, E., Evans C., and Braddick, O. J. (1983). The effects of screen size and eccentricity on acuity estimates in infants using preferential looking, *Vision Research*, 23, 1479–1483.

Atkinson, J., Braddick, O. J., Durden, K., Watson, P. G., and Atkinson, S. (1984), Screening for refractive errors in 6–9 month old infants by photorefraction. *British Journal of Ophthalmology*, 68, 105–112.

Atkinson, J., Pimm-Smith, E., Evans, C., Harding, G., and Braddick, O. J. (1986a). Visual crowding in young children. *Documenta Ophthalmologica Proceedings Series*, 45, 201–213.

Atkinson, J., Hood, B., Wattam-Bell, J., Anker, S., and Tricklebank, J. (1988b) Development of orientation discrimination in infancy. *Perception,* 17, 587–595.

Atkinson, J., Wattam-Bell, J., and Braddick, O. J. (1986b). Infants' development of sensitivity to pattern 'textons'. *Investigative Ophthalmology and Visual Science (Suppl.)*, 27, 265.

Atkinson, J., Anker, S., Evans, C., and McIntyre, A. (1987). The Cambridge Crowding Cards for preschool visual acuity testing. In *Transactions of the 6th International Orthoptic Congress*, Harrogate, UK.

Atkinson, J., Anker, S., Evans, C., Hall, R., and Pimm-Smith, E. (1988a). Visual acuity testing of young children with the Cambridge Crowding Cards at 3 and 6 metres. *Acta Ophthalmologica*, 66, 505–508.

Atkinson, J., Hood, B., Braddick, O. J., and Wattam-Bell, J. (1988b). Infants' control of fixation shifts with single and competing targets: mechanisms of shifting attention. *Perception,* 17, 367–368.

Atkinson, J., Braddick, O. J., Weeks, F., and Hood, B. (1990). Spatial and temporal tuning of infants' orientation-specific responses. *Perception,* 19, 371.

Atkinson, J., Braddick, O. J., Anker, S., Hood, B., Wattam-Bell, J., Weeks, F., Rennie J., and Coughtrey, H. (1991) Visual development in the VLBW infant. *Transactions of the 3rd Meeting of the Child Vision Research Society.* Rotterdam.

Atkinson, J., Hood, B., Wattam-Bell J., and Braddick, O. J. (1992*a*). Changes in infants' ability to switch visual attention in the first three months of life. *Perception,* 21, 643–653.

Atkinson, J., Weeks, F., Anker S., and Braddick, O. J. (1992*b*). Plasticity of orientation-selective cortical mechanisms in human infants. *Investigative Ophthalmology and Visual Science (Suppl.),* 33, 1257.

Atkinson, J., King, J., Braddick, O., Noakes, L., Anker, S., and Braddick, F. (1997). A specific deficit of dorsal stream function in Williams Syndrome. *NeuroReport,* 8, 1919–1922.

Atkinson, J., Anker, S., Ehrlich, D.,Braddick, O., Rae, S., Weeks, F., and Macpherson, J. (1995). The second Cambridge infant population screening programme using videorefraction without cycloplegia. *Strabismus,* 3, 191.

Atkinson, J., Braddick, O. J., Bobier, W., Anker, S., Ehrlich, D., King, J., Watson, P. G., and Moore, A. T. (1996). Two infant vision screening programmes: prediction and prevention of strabismus and amblyopia from photo- and videorefractive screening. *Eye,* 10, 189–198.

Atkinson, J., Braddick, O., Lin, M. H., Curran, W., Guzzetta, A., and Cioni, G. (1999). Form and motion coherence: is there a dorsal stream vulnerability in development? *Investigative Ophthalmology and Visual Science,* 40(4), S395.

Badcock, D. R. (1990). Phase- or energy-based face discrimination: Some problems. *Journal of Experimental Psychology: Human Perception and Performance,* 16, 217–220.

Baddeley, A. D. and Hitch, G. (1974). Working memory. In Bower G.H. (Ed.), *The Psychology of Learning and Motivation,* 8, 47–90

Baker, C. L., Hess, R. F., and Zihl, J. (1991). Residual motion perception in a 'motion-blind' patient, assessed with limited-lifetime random dot stimuli. *Journal of Neuroscience,* 11, 454–461.

Baldwin, W. (1990). Refractive status of infants and children. In *Principles and practice of pediatric ophthalmology,* Chapter 6. Philadelphia: Lippincott.

Banks, M. S. (1980). The development of visual accommodation during early infancy. *Child Development,* 51, 646–666.

Banks, M. S. and Bennett, P. J. (1988). Optical and photoreceptor immaturities limit the spatial and chromatic vision of human neonates. *Journal of the Optical Society of America,* A5, 2059–2079.

Baylis, G. C., Rolls, E. T., and Leonard, C. M. (1985). Selectivity between faces in the responses of a population of neurons in the cortex in the superior temporal sulcus of the monkey. *Brain Research,* 342, 91–102.

Beck, J. (1966). Effect of orientation and shape similarity on perceptual grouping. *Perception and Psychophysics,* 1, 300–2.

Bellugi, U., Sabo, H., and Vaid, J. (1988). Spatial deficits in children with Williams syndrome. In J. Stiles-Davis, M. Kritchevsky, and U. Bellugi (Eds), *Spatial cognition: brain bases and development*, pp. 273–298. Hillsdale NJ: Lawrence Erlbaum.

Bellugi, U., Bihrle A., Trauner, D., Jernigan, T., and Doherty, S. (1990). Neuropsychological, neurological, and neuroanatomical profile of Williams syndrome children. *American Journal of Medical Genetics (Suppl.)*, 6, 115–125.

Berns, G. S., Dayan P., and Sejnowski, T. J. (1993). A correlational model for the development of disparity selectivity in visual-cortex that depends on prenatal and postnatal phases. *Proceedings of the National Academy of Sciences of the USA*, 90, 8277–8281.

Bertenthal, B. I. (1993). Infants' perception of biomechanical motion: Intrinsic image and knowledge-based constraints. In C. Granrud (Ed.), *Visual perception and cognition in infancy: Carnegie-Mellon symposia on cognition* (pp. 175–214). Hillsdale, NJ: Lawrence Erlbaum Associates.

Bertenthal, B. I., Proffitt, D. R., and Cutting, J. E. (1984). Infant sensitivity to figural coherence in biomechanical motions. *Journal of Experimental Child Psychology*, 37, 213–230.

Bertenthal, B. I., Proffitt, D. R., and Kramer, S. J. (1987). Perception of biomechanical motions by infants: Implementation of various processing constraints. *Journal of Experimental Psychology; Human Perception and Performance*. 13, 577–585.

Berthoz, A. (1996). Neural basis of decision in perception and the control of movement. In A. R. Damasio, H. Damasio, and Y. Christen (Eds), *Neurobiology of decision making*. Berlin: Springer-Verlag.

Birch, E. (1993). Stereopsis in infants and its developmental relation to visual acuity. In K. Simons (Ed.), *Early visual development: normal and abnormal*. New York: Oxford University Press.

Birch, E. E. and Stager, D. R. (1985). Monocular acuity and stereopsis in infantile esotropia. *Investigative Ophthalmology and Visual Science*, 26, 1624–1630.

Birch, E. E., Gwiazda, J., and Held, R. (1982). Stereoacuity development for crossed and uncrossed disparities in human infants. *Vision Research*, 22, 507–513.

Birch, E. E., Gwiazda, J., and Held, R. (1983). The development of vergence does not account for the development of stereopsis. *Perception*, 12, 331–336.

Birch, E. E., Stager, D. R., and Wright, W. W. (1986). Grating acuity development after early surgery for congenital unilateral cataract. *Archives of Ophthalmology*, 104, 1783–1787.

Bishop, D. V. M. (1990). *Handedness and Developmental Disorder*. Hove, UK: Lawrence Erlbaum.

Blakemore, C. and Cooper, G. (1970) Development of the brain depends on the visual environment. *Nature*, 228, 477–478.

Blakemore, C. and Vital-Durand, F. (1986). Organization and postnatal development of the monkey's lateral geniculate nucleus. *Journal of Physiology. (London)*, 380, 453–491.

Boothe, R. G. (1996). Visual development following treatment of a unilateral infantile cataract. In F. Vital-Durand, O. Braddick, and J. Atkinson (Eds), *Infant vision* (pp. 401–412). Oxford University Press.

Bornstein, M. H. (1985). Habituation of attention as a measure of visual information processing in human infants: Summary, systematization, and synthesis. In G. Gottlieb and N. Krasnegor (Eds), *Measurement of audition and vision in the first year of life*. 253–300. Norwood NJ: Ablex.

Bornstein, M. H. (1998). Stability in mental development from early life: methods, measures, models, meanings and myths. In G. Butterworth and F. Simion (Eds), *The development of sensory, motor and cognitive capacities in early infancy: from perception to cognition*, pp. 301–332. Hove, UK: Erlbaum and London: Taylor and Francis.

Bornstein, M. H. and Benasich, A. A. (1986). Infant habituation: assessments of short-term reliability and individual differences at five months. *Child Development*, 57, 87–99.

Bornstein, M. H. and Ludemann, P. L. (1989). Habituation at home. *Infant Behavioural Development*, 12, 525–529.

Bornstein, M. H., Pecheux, M.-G., and Lecuyer, R. (1988). Visual habituation in human infants: Development and rearing circumstances. *Psychological Research*, 50, 130–133.

Boussaoud, D., Ungerleider, L. G., and Desimone, R. (1990). Pathways for motion analysis: cortical connections of the medial superior temporal and fundus of the superior temporal visual areas in the macaque. *Journal of Comparative Neurology*, 296, 462–495.

Bower T. G. R. (1974). *Development in Infancy*. San Francisco: Freeman.

Bower, T. G. R. (1972). Object perception in infants. *Perception*, 1, 15–30.

Bower, T. G. R. (1976). Repetitive processes in child development. *Scientific American*, 235, 38–47.

Bower, T. G. R., Broughton, J. M., and Moore, M. K. (1970). The demonstration of intention in the reaching behaviour of neonate humans. *Nature*, 228: 670–681.

Boynton, R. (1979). *Human color vision*. New York: Holt, Rinehart Winston.

Braddick, O. J. (1993). Orientation- and motion-selective mechanisms in infants. In K. Simons (Ed.), *Early visual development: normal and abnormal* (pp. 163–177). New York: Oxford University Press.

Braddick, O. (1996a). Binocularity in infancy. *Eye*, 10, 182–188.

Braddick, O. and Atkinson, J. (1984) Photorefractive techniques: Applications in testing infants and young children. *Transactions of the British College of Ophthalmic Opticians (Optometrists) First International Congress*, 2, 26–34.

Braddick, O. J. and Atkinson, J. (1988). Sensory selectivity, attentional control, and cross-channel integration in early visual development. In A. Yonas (Ed.), *20th Minnesota symposium on child psychology*, pp. 105–143. Hillsdale, NJ: Lawrence Erlbaum.

Braddick, O. J. and Atkinson, J. (1995). Visual and visuo-spatial development in young Williams syndrome children. *Investigative Ophthalmology and Visual Science (Suppl.)*, 36, S954.

Braddick, O. J., Atkinson, J., French, J., and Howland, H. C. (1979). A photorefractive study of infant accommodation. *Vision Research*, 19, 1319–1330.

Braddick, O. J., Atkinson, J., Julesz, B., Kropfl, W., Bodis-Wollner, I., and Raab, E.

(1980). Cortical binocularity in infants. *Nature,* **288,** 363–65.

Braddick, O. J., Wattam-Bell, J., Day, and Atkinson, J. (1983). The onset of binocular function in human infants. *Human Neurobiology,* **2,** 65–69.

Braddick, O. J., Wattam-Bell, J., and Atkinson, J. (1986*a*). Orientation-specific cortical responses develop in early infancy. *Nature,* **320,** 617–619.

Braddick, O. J., Atkinson, J., and Wattam-Bell, J. (1986*b*). Development of the discrimination of spatial phase in infancy. *Vision Research,* **26,** 1223–1239.

Braddick, O. J., Atkinson, J., Wattam-Bell, J., Anker, S., and Norris, V. (1988). Videorefractive screening of accommodative performance in infants. *Investigative Ophthalmology and Visual Science (Suppl.),* **29,** 60.

Braddick, O. J., Atkinson J., and Wattam-Bell, J. (1989). Development of visual cortical selectivity: binocularity, orientation, and direction of motion. In C. von Euler (Ed.), *Neurobiology of early infant behaviour* (pp. 165–172). Wenner-Gren Symposium Series, Macmillan, London.

Braddick, O., Atkinson, J., Hood, B., Harkness, W., Jackson, G., Vargha-Khadem, F. (1992). Possible blindsight in babies lacking one cerebral hemisphere. *Nature,* **360,** 461–463.

Braddick, O., Atkinson J., and Wattam-Bell, J. (1993). Infants' sensitivity to second order motion. *Strabismus,* **1,** 212.

Braddick, O. Atkinson J., and Hood, B. (1996*a*). Monocular vs binocular control of infants' reaching. *Investigative Ophthalmology and Visual Science,* **37,** S290.

Braddick, O., Atkinson, J., and Hood, B. (1996*b*). Striate cortex, extrastriate cortex, and colliculus: some new approaches. In F. Vital-Durand, O. Braddick, and J. Atkinson (Eds), *Infant vision,* pp. 203–220. Oxford University Press.

Braddick, O. J., Hartley, T., O'Brien, Atkinson, J. Wattam-Bell, J., and Turner, R. (1998*a*). Brain areas differentially activated by coherent visual motion and dynamic noise. *NeuroImage,* **7,** S322.

Braddick, O., Mercuri, E., Atkinson, J., and Wattam-Bell, J. (1998*b*). Basis of the naso-temporal asymmetry in infants' VEPs to grating displacements. *Investigative Ophthalmology and Visual Science,* **39,** S884.

Bremmer, F., Duhamel, J. -R., Ben Hamed, S., Graf, W. (1997). The representation of movement in near extra-personal space in the macaque ventral intraparietal area (VIP). In P. Thier and H.-O. Karnath (Eds) *Parietal lobe contributions to orientation in 3D space* (pp. 255–270). Heidelberg: Springer-Verlag.

Britten, K. H., Shadlen, M. N., Newsome, W. T., and Movshon, J. A. (1992). The analysis of visual motion: A comparison of neuronal and psychophysical performance. *Journal of Neuroscience,* **12,** 4745–4765.

Broadbent, D. E. (1958). *Perception and Communication.* London: The Scientific Book Guild.

Bronson, G. W. (1974). The postnatal growth of visual capacity. *Child Development,* **45,** 873–890.

Bronson, G. W. (1990). Changes in infants visual scanning across the 2- to 14-week period. *Journal of Experimental Child Psychology,* **49,** 101–125.

Brookman, K. E. (1983). Ocular accommodation in human infants. *American Journal of Optometry and Physiological in Optics,* **60,** 91–99.

Brown, A. M. (1990). Development of visual sensitivity to light and color vision in human infants: A critical review. *Vision Research*, **30**, 1159–1188.

Brown, A., Lindsey, D., McSweeney, E., and Walters, M. (1995). Infant luminance and chromatic contrast sensitivity: OKN data on 3-month olds. *Vision Research*, **35**, 3145–3160.

Bruner, J. S. (1969). On voluntary action and its hierarchical structure. *International Journal of Psychology*, **4**, 239–255.

Bruner, J. S. and Klossowski, B. (1972). Visually preadapted constituents of manipulatory action. *Perception*, **1**, 3–14.

Bushnell, E. W., McKenzie, B. E., Lawrence, D. A., and Connell, S. (1995). The spatial coding strategies of ony-year-old infants in a locomotor search task. *Child Development*, **66**, 937–958.

Bushnell, I. W. R. (1979). Modification of the externality effect in young infants. *Journal of Experimental Child Psychology*, **28**, 211–229.

Bushnell, I. W. R. (1982). Discrimination of faces by young infants. *Journal of Experimental Child Psychology*, **33**, 298–308.

Bushnell, I. W. R., Sai, F., and Mullin, J. T. (1989). Neonatal recognition of the mother's face. *British Journal of Developmental Psychology*, **7**, 3–15.

Butterworth, G., Verweij, E., and Hopkins, B. (1997). The development of prehension in infants: Halverson revisited. *British Journal of Developmental Psychology*, **15**, 223–236.

Cajal, S. R. (1909). Histologie du système nerveux de l'homme et des vertébrés. Paris: Maloine.

Campbell, F. W., and Robinson, J. G. (1968). Applications of Fourier analysis to the visibility of gratings. *Journal of Physiology*, **197**, 551–566.

Caron, A. J. and Caron, R. F. (1969). Degree of stimulus complexity and habituation of visual fixation in infants. *Psychonomic Science*, **14**, 78–79.

Cavanagh, P. and Mather, G. (1989). Motion: the long and the short of it. *Spatial Vision*, **4**, 103–29.

Charles, S. J. and Moore, A. T. (1992). Results of early surgery for infantile esotropia in normal and neurologically impaired infants. *Eye*, **6**, 603–6.

Christensen, A. M. and Wallman, J. (1991). Evidence that increased scleral growth underlies visual deprivation myopia in chicks. *Investigative Ophthalmology and Visual Science*, **32**, 2143–50.

Chubb, C. and Sperling, G. (1988). Drift-balanced random stimuli: a general basis for studying non-Fourier motion perception. *Journal of the Optical Society of America A*, **5**, 1986–2007.

Chung, S. C. and Dowling, J. E. (1997). Isolation and characterization of a motion sensitive-defective mutant in zebrafish. *Investigative Ophthalmology and Visual Science*, **38**, 2888.

Clavadetscher, J. E., Brown, A. M., Ankrum, C., and Teller, D. Y. (1988). Spectral sensitivity and chromatic discriminations in 3- and 7-week-old human infants. *Journal of the Optical Society of America A*, **5**, 2093–2105.

Colby, C. L., Duhamel, J. R., and Goldberg, M. E. (1993). Ventral intraparietal area of the macaque: anatomic location and visual response properties. *Journal of*

Neurophysiology, **69**, 902–914.

Cornelissen, P., Richardson, A., Mason, A., Fowler, S., and Stein, J. (1995). Contrast sensitivity and coherent motion detection measured at photopic luminance levels in dyslexics and controls. *Vision Research*, **35**, 1483–1494.

Craik, K. J. W. (1966). In *The nature of psychology*, Sherwood S. L. (Ed.), Cambridge: Cambridge university Press.

Crair, M. C., Gillespie, D. C., and Stryker, M. P. (1998). The role of visual experience in the development of columns in cat visual cortex. *Science*, **279**, 566–570.

Cowey, A. (1994). Cortical visual areas and the neurobiology of higher visual processes. In M. J. Farah and G. Ratcliff (Eds), *The neuropsychology of high-level vision*, pp. 3–31. Hillsdale, NJ: Lawrence Erlbaum.

Crick, F. and Koch, C. (1998). Constraints on cortical and thalamic projections: the no-strong-loops hypothesis. *Nature*, **391**, 245–250.

Crognale, M. A., Kelly, J. P., Crognale, S., Weiss, A., Teller, D. Y. (1997). Longitudinal development of the chromatic onset VEP in infants. In: *Fourteenth symposium of the international research group on colour vision deficiencies*. Ghent.

Curran, W., Braddick, O., Atkinson, J., Wattam-Bell, J., and Andrew, R. (1998). Development of illusory contour perception in infants. *Investigative Ophthalmology and Visual Science*, **39**, S884.

Curran, W., Braddick, O. J., Atkinson, J., Wattam-Bell, J., and Andrew, R. (1999). Development of illusory-contour perception in infants. *Perception*, **28**, 527–538.

Cutting, J. E. (1986). *Perception with an eye for motion*. Cambridge, MA: MIT Press.

Damasio, A. R. and Benton, A. L. (1979). Impairment of hand movements under visual guidance. *Neurology*, **29**, 170–178.

Daw, N. W. (1995). *Visual development*. New York: Plenum Press

Daw, N. W. and Wyatt, H. J. (1976). Kittens reared in a unidirectional environment: evidence for a critical period. *Journal of Physiology*, **257**, 155–170.

De Renzi, E. (1982). *Disorders of space exploration and cognition*. New York: Wiley.

Deary, I. J., Carly, P. G., Eagan, V., and Wright, D. (1989). Visual and auditory inspection time: their interrelationship and correlations with IQ in high ability subjects. *Personality and Individual Differences*, **10**, 525–533.

Derrington, A. M. and Lennie, P. (1982). The influence of temporal frequency and adaptation level on receptive-field organization of retinal ganglion-cells in cat. *Journal of Physiology*, **333**, 343–366.

Desimone, R. (1991). Face-selective cells in the temporal cortex of monkeys. *Journal of Cognitive Neursoscience*, **3**, 1–8.

Desimone, R. and Duncan, J. (1995). Neural mechanisms of selective attention. *Annual Review of Neuroscience*, **18**, 193–222.

Diamond, A., Prevor, B., Callendar, G., and Druin, D. P. (1997). Prefrontal cortex cognitive deficits in children treated early and continuously for PKU. *Monographs of the Society for Research in Child Development*. **62**, 1–207.

DiFranco, D., Muir, D. W., and Dodwell, P. C. (1978). Reaching in very young infants. *Perception*, **7**, 385–392.

Dobson, V. (1976). Spectral sensitivity of the 2-month infant as measured by the visually evoked cortical potential. *Vision Research*, **16**, 367–374.

Dobson, V. and Teller, D. Y. (1978). Visual acuity in human infants: a review and comparison of behavioral and electrophysiological studies. *Vision Research*, **18**, 1469–1483.

Dobkins, K. R., Lia, B., and Teller, D. Y. (1993). Infant color vision: Temporal contrast sensitivity functions for chromatically-defined stimuli in 3-month-olds. *Vision Research*, **37**, 1–18.

Downing, C. J. and Pinker, S. (1985). The spatial structure of visual attention. In Posner, M. I. and Marin, O. S. M. (Eds), *Attention and Performance XI*, Hillsdale, NJ: Erlbaum.

Duhamel, J. R., Bremmer, F., BenHamed, S., and Graf, W. (1997). Spatial invariance of visual receptive fields in parietal cortex neurons. *Nature*, **389**, 845–848.

Duncan, J. (1996). Cooperating brain systems in selective perception and action. In *Attention and performance XVI*. Inui T. and McClelland J. L. (Eds), 549–578, Cambridge, MA: MIT Press.

Dziurawiec, S. and Ellis, H. D. (1986). Neonates' attention to face-like stimuli: Goren, Sarty and Wu (1975) revisited. *Annual Conference of the British Psychological Society Developmental Section, Exeter, September 1986*.

Eden, G. F., Vanmeter, J. W., Rumsey, J. M., Maisog, J. M., Woods, R. P., and Zeffiro, T. A. (1996). Abnormal processing of visual motion in dyslexia revealed by functional brain imaging. *Nature*, **382**, 66–69.

Edwards, A. D., Wyatt, J. S., and Thoresen, M. (1998). Treatment of hypoxic-ischaemic brain damage by moderate hypothermia. *Archives of Disease in Childhood*, **78**, F85–F88.

Ehrlich, D. L., Atkinson, J., Braddick, O. J., Bobier, W., and Durden, K. (1995). Reduction of infant myopia: A longitudinal cycloplegic study. *Vision Research*, **35**, 1313–1324.

Ehrlich, D., Anker, S., Atkinson, J., Braddick, O. J., Weeks F., and Wade, J. (1996) Changes of infant refraction with age. *Investigative Ophthalmology and Visual Science*, **37**, S730.

Ehrlich, D., Braddick, O. J., Atkinson, J., Weeks, F., Hartley, T., Anker, S., Wade, J., and Rudenski, A. (1997). Infant emmetropization analysed by refractive decomposition. *Investigative Opthalmology & Visual Science*, **38**, S980.

Ewert, A. K., Morris, C. A., Atkinson, D., Jin, W. Sternes, K. Spallone, P., Stock, A. D., Leppert, M., and Keating, M. T. (1993). Hemizygosity at the elastin locus in a developmental disorder, Williams syndrome. *Nature Genetics*, **5**, 11–16.

Eyre, J. A., Miller, S., and Ranesh, V. (1991). Constancy of central conduction delays during development in man: Investigation of motor and somatosensory pathways. *Journal of Physiology*, **434**, 441–452.

Fantz, R. L., Ordy, J. M., and Udelf, M. S. (1962). Maturation of pattern vision in infants during the first six months. *Journal of Comparative and Physiological Psychology*, **55**, 907–917.

Farah, M. J. (1994). Specialization within visual object recognition. In M. J. Farah and G. Ratcliff (eds.) *The neuropsychology of high-level vision* (pp. 133–146). Hillsdale, NJ: Lawrence Erlbaum.

Fielder, A. R., Foreman, N., Moseley, M., and Robinson, J. (1993). Prematurity and visual development. In K. Simons (Ed.), *Early visual development: normal and abnormal* (pp. 485–504). New York: Oxford University Press.

Finlay, D. C. and Ivinski, A. (1984). Cardiac and visual responses to moving stimuli presented either successively or simultaneously to the central and peripheral visual fields. *Developmental Psychology*, **20**, 29–36.

Fischer, B. (1986). The role of attention in the preparation of visually guided eye movements in monkey and man. *Psychological Research,* **48**, 251–257.

Foreman, N., Fielder, A., Price, D., and Bowler, V. (1991). Tonic and phasic orientation in full-term and preterm infants. *Journal of Experimental Child Psychology*, **51**, 407–422.

Forssberg, H., Kinoshita, H., Eliasson, A. C., Johanssen, R. S., Westling, G., and Gordon, A. M. (1991). Development of precision grip I. Basic co-ordination of forces. *Experimental Brain Research*, **90**, 393–398.

Fox, R., Aslin, R. N., Shea, S. L., and Dumais, S. T. (1980). Stereopsis in human infants. *Science*, **207**, 323–324.

Frangiskakis, J. M., Ewart, A. K., Morris, C. A., Mervis, C. B., Bertrand, J., Robinson, B. F., *et al.* (1996). LIM-kinase1 hemizygosity implicated in impaired visuospatial constructive cognition. *Cell*, **86**, 59–69.

Friede, R. L. and Hu, K. H. (1967) Proximo-distal differences in myelin development in human optic fibres. *Zeitscchrift für Zellforschung*, **79**, 259–264.

Gallant, J. L., Braun, J., and Van Essen D. C. (1993) Selectivity for polar, hyperbolic, and cartesian gratings in macaque visual-cortex. *Science*, **259**, 100–103.

Garey, L. and De Courten, C. (1983). Structural development of the lateral geniculate nucleus and visual cortex in monkey and man. *Behavioural Brain Research*, **10**, 3–15.

Gauthier, G. M., Vercher, J. L., Mussa-Ivaldi, F., and Marchetti, E. (1988). Oculomanual tracing of visual targets: control learning, co-ordination control and co-ordination model. *Experimental Brain Research*, **73**, 127–137.

Gentillucci, M. and Rizzolatti, G. (1990). Cortical control of arm and hand movements. In M. A. Goodale (Ed.), *Vision and action.* pp. 147–162. New York: Ablex.

Ghim, H. (1990). Evidence for perceptual organization in infants: perception of subjective contours by young infants. *Infant Behavior and Development*, **13**, 221–248.

Ghim, H. and Eimas, P. D. (1988). Global and local processing by 3- and 4-month-old infants. *Perception and Psychophysics*, **43**, 165–171.

Gibson, J. J. (1950). *The perception of the visual world.* New York: Appleton-Century-Crofts.

Glickstein, M. and May, J. G. (1982). In: W. D. Neff (Ed.), *Contributions to sensory physiology* Vol. 7. New York: Academic Press.

Goren, C. C., Sarty, M., and Wu, P. Y. K. (1975). Visual following and visual discrimination of face-like stimuli by newborn infants. *Pediatrics*, **56**, 544–549.

Granrud, C. E. (1986). Binocular vision and spatial perception in 4- and 5-month-old infants. *Journal of Experimental Psychology: Human Perception and Performance*, **12**, 36–49.

Grosof, D., Shapley, R. M., and Hawken, M. J. (1993). Macaque V1 neurons can signal 'illusory' contours. *Nature*, **365**, 550–552.

Grossberg, S. and Mingolla, E. (1985). Neural dynamics of form perception: Boundary completion, illusory figures, and neon color spreading. *Psychological Review*, 92, 173–211.

Guillery, R. W. (1996). The reasons for the loss of binocularity in albinism. *Eye*, 10, 217–221.

Gwiazda, J., Bauer, J., Thorn, F., and Held, R. (1986). Meridional amblyopia *does* result from astigmatism in early childhood. *Clinical Vision Sciences*, 1, 145–152.

Haddersalgra, M. and Prechtl, H. F. R. (1992). Developmental course of general movements in early infancy. 1. Descriptive analysis of change in form. *Early Human Development*, 28, 201–213.

de Haan, M., Johnson, M. H., and Maurer, D. (1998). Recognition of individual faces and average face prototypes by 1- and 30-month infants. *Developmental Cognitive Neuroscience Technical Report no. 98. 8*: Centre for Brain and Cognitive Development, Birkbeck College.

de Haan, M., Oliver, A., and Johnson, M. H. (in press). Spatial and temporal characteristics of electro-cortical activation in adults and infants viewing faces. *Journal of Neuroscience.*

Hainline, L. (1985). Oculomotor control in human infants. In R. Groner, G. W. McConkie, and C. Menz (Eds), *Eye movements and human information processing*, pp. 71–84. Elsevier-North Holland: Amsterdam.

Hainline, L. (1993). Conjugate eye movements of infants. In K. Simons (Ed.), *Early visual development: normal and abnormal*, pp. 47–79. New York: Oxford University Press.

Hainline, L. and Riddell, P. M. (1995). Binocular alignment and vergence in early infancy. *Vision Research*, 35, 3229–3236.

Hainline, L. and Riddell, P. (1996). Eye alignment and convergence in young infants. In F. Vital-Durand, O. Braddick, and J. Atkinson (Eds), *Infant vision*, pp. 221–248. Oxford University Press.

Hainline, L., Turkel, J., Abramov, I., Lemerise, E., and Harris, C. (1984). Characteristics of saccades in human infants. *Vision Research*, 24, 1771–1780.

Hainline, L., Riddell, P., Grose-Fifer, J., and Abramov, I. (1992). Development of accommodation and convergence in infancy. *Behavioural Brain Research*, 49, 33–50.

Haith, M. M., Bergman, T., and Moore, M. J. (1977). Eye contact and early scanning in early infancy. *Science*, 198, 853–855.

Halverson, H. M. (1937). Studies of grasping responses in early infancy. *Journal of Genetic Psychology*, 7, 34–63.

Hamer, R. D., Alexander, K. R., and Teller, D. Y. (1982). Rayleigh discriminations in young human infants. *Vision Research*, 22, 575–587.

Harris, L., Atkinson J., and Braddick, O. J. (1976). Visual contrast sensitivity of a 6-month infant measured by the evoked potential. *Nature*, 264, 570–571.

Harris, P. and MacFarlane, A. (1974). The growth of the effective visual field from birth to seven weeks. *Journal of Experimental Child Psychology*, 18, 340–348.

Hayhoe, M. and Land, M. (1999). Coordination of eye and hand movements in a normal visual environment. *Investigative Ophthalmology and Visual Science*, 40, S380.

Hein, A. and Held, R. (1967). Dissociation of the visual placing response into elicited and guided components. *Science*, **158**, 190–192.

Held, R. (1979). Development of visual resolution. *Canadian Journal of Psychology*, **33**, 213–221.

Held, R. (1993). Two stages in the development of binocular vision and eye alignment. In K. Simons (Ed.), *Early visual development: normal and abnormal*, 250–257. New York: Oxford University Press.

Held, R., Birch, E. E., and Gwiazda J. (1980). Stereoacuity of human infants. *Proceedings of the National Academy of Sciences of the USA*, **77**, 5572–5574.

Hermer, L. and Spelke, E. S. (1994). A geometric process for spatial reorientation in young children. *Nature*, **370**, 57–59.

Hermer, L. and Spelke, E. S. (1996). Modularity and development: The case of spatial reorientation. *Cognition*, **61**, 195–232.

Hess, R. F., Campbell, F. W., and Greenhalgh, T. (1978). On the nature of the neural abnormality in human myoblopia: Neural abberations and neural sensitivity loss. *Pflügers Archiv Gesamte Physiologie*, **377** 201–207.

von der Heydt, R. and Peterhans, E. (1989). Mechanisms of contour perception in monkey visual cortex. *Journal of Neuroscience*, **9**, 1731–1748.

von der Heydt, R., Peterhans, E., and Baumgartner, M. (1984). Illusory contours and cortical neurone responses. *Science*, **224**, 1260–1262.

Hickey, T. L. and Peduzzi, J. D. (1987). Structure and development of the visual system. In P. Salapatek and L. B. Cohen (Eds), *Handbook of infant perception* (pp. 1–42). New York: Academic Press.

Hirsch, H. and Spinelli, D. (1970). Visual experience modifies distribution of horizontally and vertically oriented receptive fields in cat. *Science*, **168**, 869–871.

Hoffmann K-P (1981). Neuronal responses related to optokinetic nystagmus in the cat's nucleus of the optic tract. In A. Fuchs and W. Becker (Eds), *Progress in oculomotor research* (pp. 443–454). New York: Elsevier.

von Hofsten, C. (1979). Development of visually guided reaching: the approach phase. *Journal of Motor Behaviour*, **5**, 160–178.

von Hofsten, C. (1982). Eye-hand coordination in newborns. *Developmental Psychology*, **18**, 450–461.

von Hofsten, C. (1984). Developmental changes in the organization of pre-reaching. *Developmental Psychology*, **18**, 450–461.

von Hofsten, C. (1991). Structuring of early reaching movements: a longitudinal study. *Journal of Motor Behaviour*, **23**, 280–292.

von Hofsten, C. and Fazel-Dandy, S. (1984). Development of visually guided hand orientation in reaching. *Journal of Experimental Child Psychology*, **38**, 208–219.

von Hofsten, C. and Ronqvist, L. (1988). Preparation for grasping an object: a developmental study. *Journal of Experimental Psychology: Human Perception and Performance*, **14**, 610–621.

Hood, B. (1991). Development of visual selective attention in the human infant. PhD thesis, University of Cambridge.

Hood, B. (1993). Inhibition of return produced by covert shifts of visual attention in 6 month-old infants. *Infant Behaviour and Development,* **16**, 255–264.

Hood, B. and Atkinson, J. (1990). Sensory visual loss and cognitive deficits in the selective attentional system of normal infants and neurologically impaired children. *Developmental Medicine and Child Neurology*, 32, 1067–1077.

Hood, B. and Atkinson, J. (1991). Shifting covert attention in infants. *Investigative Ophthalmology and Visual Science (Suppl.)*, 32, 965.

Hood, B. and Atkinson, J. (1993) Disengaging visual attention in the infant and adult. *Infant Behaviour and Development*, 16, 405–422.

Hood, B., Murray, L., King, F., Hooper, R., Atkinson, J., and Braddick, O. J. (1994). Longitudinal measures of habituation from birth to six months. *Infant Behaviour and Development*, 17, 715.

Horowitz, F. D., Paden, L., Bhana, K., and Self, P. (1972). An infant-controlled procedure for studying infant visual fixations. *Developmental Psychology*, 7, 90.

Horton, J. C. and Hedley-White, T. (1984). Mapping of cytochrome oxidase patches and ocular dominance columns in human visual cortex. *Philosophical Transactions of the Royal Society of London B*, 304, 252–272.

Howland, H. C. (1993). Early refractive development. In K. Simons (Ed.), *Early visual development: normal and abnormal*, pp. 5–31. New York: Oxford University Press.

Howland, H. C. and Howland, B. (1974). Photorefraction, a technique for the study of refractive state at a distance. *Journal of the Optical Society of America*, 64, 240–249.

Howland, H. C., Atkinson, J., Braddick, O. J., and French, J. (1978). Infant astigmatism measured by photorefraction. *Science*, 202, 331–333.

Howland, H. C., Braddick, O. J., Atkinson, J., and Howland, B. (1983). Optics of photorefraction: orthogonal and isotropic methods. *Journal of the Optical Society of America*, 73, 1701–1708.

Howland, H. C., Dobson, V., and Sayles, N. (1987). Accommodation in infants as measured by photorefraction. *Vision Research*, 27, 2141–2152.

Hubel, D. H. and Wiesel, T. N. (1977). Functional architecture of macaque monkey visual cortex. *Proceedings of the Royal Society of London B*, 198, 1–59.

Hung, L. F., Crawford, M. L. J., and Smith, E. L. (1995). Spectacle lenses alter eye growth and the refractive status of young monkeys. *Nature Medicine*, 1, 761–765.

Huttenlocher, P. R., de Courten, C., Garey, L. G., and van der Loos, H. (1982). Synaptogenesis in human visual cortex—evidence for synapse elimination during normal development. *Neuroscience Letters*, 33, 247–252.

Jacobs, D. S. and Blakemore, C. (1988). Factors limiting the postnatal development of visual acuity in the monkey. *Vision Research*, 28, 947–958.

Jeannerod, M. (1986). Mechanisms of visuomotor co-ordination. A study in normal and brain-damaged patients. *Neuropsychologia*, 24, 41–78.

Jeannerod, M. (1988). *The neural and behavioural organization of goal directed movements*. Oxford: Oxford University Press.

Jeannerod, M. (1997). *The cognitive neuroscience of action*. Oxford: Blackwell.

Jernigan, T. L., Bellugi, U., Sowell, E., Doherty, S., and Hesselink, J. R. (1993). Cerebral morphologic distinctions between Williams and Down syndromes. *Archives of Neurology*, 50, 186–191.

Johansson, G. (1975). Visual motion perception. *Scientific American*, **232**(6), 76–88.

Johnson, C. A., Post, R. B., Chalupa, L. M., and Lee, T. J. (1982). Monocular deprivation in humans: a study of identical twins. *Investigative Ophthalmology and Visual Science*, **23**, 135–140.

Johnson, M. H. (1990). Cortical maturation and the development of visual attention in early infancy. *Journal of Cognitive Neuroscience*, **2**, 81–95.

Johnson, M. H. and Tucker, L. A. (1993). The ontogeny of covert visual attention: facilitatory and inhibitory effects. *Abstracts of the Society for Research in Child Development*, **9**, 24.

Johnson, M. H., Posner, M. I., and Rothbart, M. K. (1991). Components of visual orienting in early infancy: contingency learning, anticipatory looking, and disengaging. *Journal of Cognitive Neuroscience*, **3**, 336–344.

Johnson, S. P. (1998). Object perception and object knowledge in young infants: A view from studies of visual development. In A. Slater (ed.), *Perceptual Development: Visual, Auditory, and Speech Perception in Infancy*, pp. 211–239. Hove, England: Psychology Press.

Judge, S. J. (1996). How is binocularity maintained during convergence and divergence? *Eye*, **10**, 172–176.

Julesz, B. (1981). Textons, the elements of texture perception, and their interactions. *Nature*, **290**, 91–97.

Julesz, B., Kropfl, W., and Petrig, B. (1980). Large evoked potentials of dynamic random-dot correlograms and stereograms permit quick determination of stereopsis. *Proceedings of the National Academy of Sciences of the USA*, **77**, 2348–2351.

Kanwisher, N., McDermott, J., and Chun, M. (1997). The fusiform face area: a module in human extrastriate cortex specialized for face perception. *Journal of Neuroscience*, **17**, 4302–4311.

Kellman, P. J. and Arterberry, M. E. (1998). *The cradle of knowledge*. Cambridge, MA: MIT Press.

Kellman, P. J., Gleitman, H. and Spelke, E. S. (1987). Object and observer motion in the perception of objects by human infants. *Journal of Experimental Psychology, Human Perception and Performance*, **13**, 586–593.

King, J. A. (1998). Visuomotor control in normal infants and children with Williams syndrome. PhD. thesis, University College London.

King, J. A., Atkinson, J., Braddick, O. J., Nokes, L., and Braddick, F. (1996). Target preference and movement kinematics reflect development of visuomotor modules in the reaching of human infants. *Investigative Ophthalmology and Visual Science*, **37**, S526.

King, J. A., Newman, C., Atkinson, J., Braddick, O. J., Mason, A. J. S., and Curran, W. (1998). Preferential looking and preferential reaching in infants: neurobiological models of dorsal stream development. *Perception*, **27**, S201.

Kiorpes, L. and Wallman, J. (1995). Does experimentally induced myopia cause hyperopia in monkeys? *Vision Research*, **35**, 1289–1297.

Kleiner, K. A. (1987). Amplitude and phase spectra as indices of infants' pattern preferences. *Infant Behavior and Development*, **10**, 49–59.

Koffka, K. (1935). *Principles of gestalt psychology*. New York: Harcourt, Brace and World.

Konczak, J. and Dichgans, J. (1997). The development towards stereotypic arm movements during reaching in the first three years of life. *Experimental Brain Research*, 117, 346–354.

Konczak, J. and Thelen, E. (1994). The dynamics of goal-directed reaching: a comparison of adult and infant movement patterns. In J. H. A. van Rossum and J. H. Laszlo (Eds), *Motor development: aspects of normal and delayed development* (pp. 25–40). Amsterdam: VU University Press.

Kuypers, H. G. J. M. (1962). Corticospinal connections: postnatal development in the rhesus monkey. *Science*, 138, 678–680.

LaBerge, D. and Brown, V. (1989). Theory of attentional operations in shape identification. *Psychological Review*, 96, 101–124.

Lawrence D. G. and Kuypers, H. G. J. M (1968). Functional organization of the motor system in the monkey: I. Effects of bilateral pyramidal lesions. *Brain*, 91, 1–14.

Ledgeway, T. and Smith, A. T. (1994). Evidence for separate mechanisms for first-order and second-order motion in human vision. *Vision Research*, 34, 2727–2740.

Lennie, P. (1984). Recent developments in the physiology of color vision. *Trends in Neurosciences*, 7, 243–248.

LeVay, S., Stryker, M. P., and Sherk, H. (1978). Ocular dominance columns and their development in layer IV of the cat's visual cortex: a quantitative study. *Journal of Comparative Neurology*, 179, 223–244.

Lewis, T. L., Maurer, D., and Brent, H. P. (1995). Development of grating acuity in children treated for unilateral or bilateral congenital cataract. *Investigative Ophthalmology and Visual Science,* 36, 2080–2095.

Livingstone, M. and Hubel, D. H. (1988). Segregation of form, color, movement and depth: anatomy, physiology and perception. *Science*, 240, 740–749.

Livingstone, M. S., Rosen, G. D., Drislane, F. W., and Galaburda, A. M. (1991). Physiological and anatomical evidence for a magnocellular defect in developmental dyslexia. *Proceedings of the National Academy of Sciences of USA*, 88, 7943–7947.

Lockman, J. J., Ashmead,D. H., and Bushnell, E. W. (1984). The development of anticipatory hand orientation during infancy. *Journal of Experimental Child Psychology*, 37, 176–186.

McCall, R. B. and Carriger, M. S. (1993). A meta–analysis of infant habituation and recognition memory performance as predictors of later IQ. *Child Development*, 64, 57–79.

McDonald, M. A., Sebris, S. L., Mohn, G., Teller, D. Y., and Dobson, V. (1985). The acuity card procedure: A rapid test of infant acuity. *Investigative Ophthalmology and Visual Science*, 26, 1158–1162.

McDonnell, P. M. (1975). The development of visually guided reaching. *Perception and Psychophysics*, 18, 181–185.

MacFarlane, A., Harris, P., and Barnes, I. (1976) Central and peripheral vision in early infancy. *Journal of Experimental Child Psychology*, 21, 532–538.

Marr, D. (1982). *Vision*. San Francisco: W. H. Freeman.

Mash, C., Dobson, V., and Carpenter, N. (1995). Interobserver agreement for measurement of grating acuity and interocular acuity differences with the Teller Acuity Card procedure. *Vision Research*, 35, 303–312.

Mason, A., Braddick, O., Wattam-Bell, J., and Atkinson, J. (1998). Directional motion asymmetry in infant VEPs—which direction? *Investigative Ophthalmology and Visual Science*, 39, S1090.

Mather, G. and West, S. (1993). Evidence for second-order motion detectors. *Vision Research*, 33, 1109–1112.

Mathew, A. and Cook, M. (1990). The control of reaching movements in young infants. *Child Development*, 61, 1238–1257.

Maunsell, J. H. R. and Newsome, W. T. (1987) Visual processing in monkey extrastriate cortex. *Annual Review of Neuroscience*, 10, 363–401.

Maurer, D. (1985). Infants' perception of faceness. In T. N. Field and N. Fox (Eds), *Social perception in infants* (pp. 73–100). Norwood, NJ: Ablex.

Mayer, D. L. and Dobson, V. (1980). Assessment of vision in young children: A new operant approach yields estimates of acuity. *Investigative Ophthalmology and Visual Science*, 19, 566–570.

Maurer, D. and Lewis, T. L. (1993). Visual outcomes after infantile cataract. In K. Simons (Ed.), *Early visual development: normal and abnormal* (pp. 454–484). New York: Oxford University Press.

Maurer, D. and Salapatek, P. (1976). Developmental changes in the scanning of faces by young infants. *Child Development*, 47, 523–527.

Maurer, D., Lewis, T.L., Brent, H.P., and Levin, A.V. (1999). Rapid improvement in the acuity of infants after visual input. *Science*, 286, 108–110.

Maurer, D., Lewis, T., Cavanagh, P., and Anstis, S. (1989). A new test of luminous efficiency for babies. *Investigative Ophthalmology and Visual Science*. 30, 297–303.

Mayes, L. C. Kessen, W. (1989). Maturational changes in measures of habituation. *Infant Behavior and Development,* 12, 437–450.

Mercuri, E., Atkinson, J., Braddick, O., Anker, S., Nokes, L. Cowan, F., *et al.* (1995). Visual maturation in children with focal brain lesions on neonatal imaging. *Neuropediatrics*, 26, 348.

Mercuri, E., Atkinson, J., Braddick, O., Anker, S., Nokes, L. Cowan, F., *et al.* (1996). Visual function and perinatal focal cerebral infarction. *Archives of Disease in Childhood*, 75, F76–F81.

Mercuri, E., Atkinson, J., Braddick, O., Anker, S., Nokes, L. Cowan, F., *et al.* (1997*a*). Basal ganglia damage in the newborn infant as a predictor of impaired visual function. *Archives of Disease in Childhood*, 77, F111–F114.

Mercuri, E., Atkinson, J., Braddick, O., Anker, S., Cowan, F., Rutherford, M., *et al.* (1997*b*). Visual function in full term infants with hypoxic-ischaemic encephalopathy. *Neuropediatrics* 28, 155–161.

Mercuri, E., Atkinson, J., Braddick, O., Rutherford, M., Cowan, F., Counsell, S., *et al.* (1997*c*). Chiari I malformation and white matter changes in asymptomatic young children with Williams syndrome: clinical and MRI study. *European Journal of Paediatric Neurology*, 5/6, 177–181.

Merigan, W. H. and Maunsell, J. H. R. (1993). How parallel are the primate visual pathways? *Annual Review of Neuroscience*, 16, 369–402.

Michotte, A., Thines, G., and Crabbe, G. (1964). Les complements amodaux des structures perceptives. *Studia psychologica*. Louvain: Publications Universitaire de Louvain.

Milewski, A. (1976). Infants' discrimination of internal and external pattern elements. *Journal of Experimental Child Psychology*, 22, 229–246.

Milner A. D. and Goodale, M. A. (1995). *The visual brain in action*. Oxford University Press.

Mishkin, M., Ungerleider, L., and Macko, K. A. (1983). Object vision and spatial vision: two cortical pathways. *Trends in Neuroscience*, 6, 414–417.

Mitchell, D. E., Freeman, R. D., Millodot, M., and Haegerstrom, G. (1973). Meridional amblyopia: evidence for modification of the human visual system by early visual experience. *Vision Research*, 13, 535–538.

Mohindra I., Held R., Gwiazda J., and Brill S. (1978). Astigmatism in infants. *Science*, 202, 329–31.

Mohn, G. (1989). The development of binocular and monocular optokinetic nystagmus in human infants. *Investigative Ophthalmology and Visual Science (Suppl.)*, 40, 49.

Moore, B. R. (1980). A modification of the Rayleigh test for vector data. *Biometrika*, 67, 175–180.

Morrone, M. C., Burr, D. C., and Fiorentini, A. (1990). Development of infant contrast sensitivity and acuity to chromatic stimuli. *Proceedings of the Royal Society of London B*, 242, 134–139.

Morrone, M. C., Burr, D. C., and Fiorentini, A. (1993) Development of infant contrast sensitivity to chromatic stimuli. *Vision Research*, 33, 2535–2552.

Morrone, M. C., Atkinson, J., Cioni, G., Braddick, O. J., and Fiorentini, A. (1999). Development changes in optokinetic mechanisms in the absence of unilateral cortical control. *NeuroReport*, 10, 2723–2729.

Morton, J. and Johnson, M. H. (1991). CONSPEC and CONLERN: A two-process theory of infant face recognition. *Psychological Review*, 98, 164–181.

Mounoud, P. and Vintner, A. (1981). Tire-a-part: Representation and sensorimotor development. In G. Butterworth (Ed.), *Infancy and epistemology: an evaluation of Piaget's theory*. Brighton: Harverster Press.

Mountcastle, V. B. (1978). Brain mechanisms for directed attention. *Journal of the Royal Society of Medicine*, 71, 14–28.

Movshon J. A., Adelson, E. H., Gizzi, M. S., and Newsome, W. T. (1985). The analysis of moving visual patterns. In C. Chagas, R. Gattass, and C. G. Gross (Eds), *Pattern recognition mechanisms. Pontificae Academiae Scientiarum Scripta Varia*, 54, 117–151. Vatican City: Pontifica Academia Scientiarum.

Nelson, C. A. (1994). Neural correlates of recognition memory in the first potential year of life. In Dawson G., and Fischer K. (Eds) *Human Behaviour and the Developing Brain*, 269–313. New York: Guildford Press.

Nelson, C. A. and Ludemann, P. M. (1989). Past, current, and future trends in infant face perception research. *Canadian Journal of Psychology*, 43, 183–198.

Newsome, W. T. and Paré, E. B. (1988). A selective impairment of motion processing following lesions of the middle temporal area (MT). *Journal of Neuroscience*, **8**, 2201–2211.

Norcia, A. M. (1996). Abnormal motion processing and binocularity: infantile esotropia as a model system for effects of early interruptions of binocularity. *Eye*, **10**, 259–265.

Norcia, A. M. and Tyler, C. W. (1985). Spatial frequency sweep VEP: Visual acuity during the first year of life. *Vision Research*. **25**, 1399–1408.

Norcia A. M., Hamer R. D., and Orel-Bixler D. (1990). Temporal tuning of the motion VEP in infants. *Investigative Ophthalmology and Visual Science (Suppl.)*, **31**, 10.

Norcia A. M., Garcia H., Humphry R., Holmes A., Hamer R. D., and Orel-Bixler D. (1991). Anomalous motion VEPs in infants and in infantile esotropia. *Investigative Ophthalmology and Visual Science*, **32**, 346–439.

Nothdurft, H. C. (1990). Texton segregation by associated differences in global and local luminance distribution. *Proceedings of the Royal Society of London B*, **239**, 295–320.

Olson, R. and Attneave, F. (1970). What variables produce similarity grouping? *American Journal of Psychology*, **83**, 1–21.

Packer, O., Hartmann, E. E., and Teller, D. Y. (1984). Infant color vision: the effect of field size on Rayleigh discriminations. *Vision Research*. **24**, 1247–1260.

Pascalis, O., de Schonen, S., Morton, J., Deruelle, C., and Fabre-Grenet, M. (1995). Mother's face recognition by neonates: A replication and extension. *Infant Behavior and Development*, **18**, 79–85.

Peeples, D. and Teller, D. Y. (1975). Color vision and brightness discrimination in two-month-old human infants. *Science*, **189**, 1102–1103.

Penrice, J., Cady, E. B., Lorek, A., Wylezinska, M., Amess, P. N., Aldridge, R. F., *et al.* (1996). Proton magnetic resonance spectroscopy of the brain in normal preterm and term infants, and early changes after perinatal hypoxia-ischemia. *Pediatric Research*, **40**, 6–14.

Perenin, M. T. (1978). Visual function within the hemianopic field following early cerebral hemidecortication in man—II. Pattern discrimination. *Neuropsychologia*, **16**, 697–708.

Perenin, M. T. and Jeannerod, M. (1978). Visual function within the hemianopic field following early cerebral hemidecortication in man—I. Spatial localization. *Neuropsychologia*, **16**, 1–13.

Piaget, J. (1953). *The origins of intelligence in the child*. New York: Routledge.

Pöppel, E., Held, R., and Frost, D. (1973). Residual visual function after brain wounds involving the central visual pathways in man. *Nature (London)*, **243**, 295–296.

Posner, M. I. (1980). Orienting of attention. *Quarterly Journal of Experimental Psychology*, **32**, 3–25.

Posner, M. I. and Dehaene, S. (1994). Attentional networks. *Trends in Neurosciences*, **17**, 75–79.

Posner, M. A. and Petersen, S. E. (1990). The attention system of the human brain. *Annual Review of Neuroscience*, **13**, 25–42.

Posner, M. I., Rafal, R. D., Choate, L. S., and Vaughan, J. (1985). Inhibition of return: neural basis and function. *Cognitive Neuropsychology*, **2**, 211–228.

Ptito, A., Lassonde, M., Leporé, F., and Ptito, M. (1987). Visual discrimination in hemispherectomised patients. *Neuropsychologia*, 25, 869–879.

Pulos, E., Teller, D. Y., and Buck, S. (1980). Infant color vision: a search for short wavelength-sensitive mechanisms by means of chromatic adaptation. *Vision Research*, 20, 485–493.

Provine, R. R. and Westerman, J. A. (1979). Crossing the midline: limits of early eye-hand behaviour. *Child Development*, 50, 437–441.

Prechtl, H. F. R. (1974). The behavioural states of the newborn infant (a review). *Brain Research*, 76, 185–212.

Rada, J. A., Thoft, R. A., and Hassell, J. R. (1991). Increased aggrecan (cartilage protoglycan) production in the sclera of myopic chick. *Developmental Biology*, 147, 303–312.

Rader, N. and Stern, J. D. (1982). Visually elicited reaching in neonates. *Child Development*, 53, 1004–1007.

Rafal, R., Calabresi, P., Brennan, C., and Sciolto, T. (1989). Saccade preparation inhibits reorienting to recently attended locations. *Journal of Experimental Psychology: Human Perception and Performance*, 15, 673–685.

Rafal, R., Henkin, A., and Smith, J. (1991). Extrageniculate contributions to reflex visual orienting in normal humans—a temporal hemifield advantage. *Journal of Cognitive Neuroscience*, 3(4), 322–328.

Rakic, P. (1977). Prenatal development of the visual system in rhesus monkey. *Philosophical Transactions of the Royal Society of London B*, 278, 245–260.

Rauschecker, J. P. and Singer, W. (1981) The effects of early visual experience on the cat's visual cortex and their possible explanation by Hebb synapses. *Journal of Physiology*, 310, 215–239.

Regan, D. (1989). *Human brain electrophysiology: evoked potentials and evoked magnetic fields in science and medicine*. New York: Elsevier.

Richards, J. E. (1989). Development and stability of visual sustained attention in 14, 20, and 26 week old infants. *Psychophysiology*, 26, 422–430.

Richards, J. E. and Casey, B. J. (1992). Development of sustained visual attention in the human infant. In B. A. Campbell, H. Hayne, and R. Richardson (Eds) *Attention and information processing in infants and adults* (pp. 30–60). Hillsdale, NJ: Lawrence Erlbaum.

Rieth, C and Sireteanu, R. (1994). Texture segmentation and 'pop-out' in infants and children: A study with the forced-choice preferential looking method. *Spatial Vision*, 8, 173–191.

Rizzolatti, G. (1983). Mechanisms of selective attention in mammals. In J.-P. Ewwert, R. Capranica, and D. J. Ingle (Eds), *Advances in vertebrate neuroethology* (pp. 261–297). Amsterdam: Elsevier.

Rizzolatti, G. and Camarda, R. (1987). Neural circuits for spatial attention and unilateral neglect. In M. Jeannerod (Ed.), *Neurophysiological and neuropsychological aspects of spatial neglect* (pp. 289–213). Amsterdam: Elsevier.

Rizzolatti, G., Riggio, L., Dascola, I., and Umilta, C. (1987). Reorienting attention across the horizontal and vertical meridians: evidence in favour of a premotor theory of attention. *Neuropsychologia*, 25, 31–40.

Rizzolatti, G., Fogassi, L., and Gallese, V. (1997). Parietal cortex: from sight to action. *Current Opinion in Neurobiology*, 7, 562–567.

Rochat, P. (1992). Self-sitting and reaching in 5- to 8-month-old infants: The impact of posture and its development on early eye-hand co-ordination. *Journal of Motor Behaviour*, 24, 210–220.

Rodman, H. R., Gross, C. G., and Scalaidhe, S. P. (1993). Development of brain substrates for pattern recognition in primates: physiological and connectional studies of inferior temporal cortex in infant monkeys. In B. de Boysson-Bardies, S. de Schonen, P. Jusczyk, P. McNeilage, and J. Morton (Eds), *Developmental neurocognition: speech and face processing in the first year of life* (pp. 63–76). Kluwer: Dordrecht.

Ruff, H. A. and Halton, A. (1978). Is there directed reaching in the human neonate? *Developmental Psychology*, 14, 425–426.

Sagi, D. and Julesz, B (1985) 'Where' and 'what' in vision. *Science*, 228, 1217–1219.

Sakata, H. Taira, M., Mine, S., and Murata, A. (1992). Hand-movement related neurons of the posterior parietal cortex of the monkey: their role in visual guidance of hand movements. In R. Caminiti, P. B. Johnson, and Y. Burnod (Eds), *Control of arm movement in space: neurophysiological and computational approaches* (pp. 185–198). Heidelberg: Springer-Verlag.

Salapatek, P. (1975). Pattern perception in early infancy. In L. B. Cohen and P. Salapatek (Eds), *Infant perception: from sensation to cognition*, Vol. I, pp. 133–248. New York: Academic Press.

Salt, A. T., Sonksen, P. M., Wade, A., and Jayatunga, R. (1995). The maturation of linear acuity and compliance with the Sonksen-Silver Acuity System in young children. *Developmental Medicine & Child Neurology*. 37, 505–514.

Sarnat, H. B. and Sarnat, M. S. (1976). Neonatal encephalopathy following fetal distress: A clinical and electrophysiological study. *Archives of Neurology*, 33, 696–705.

Saslow, M. G. (1967). Effects of components of displacement-step stimuli upon latency of saccadic eye movements. *Journal of the Optical Society of America*, 57, 1024–1029.

Scase, M. O., Braddick, O. J., and Raymond, J. E. (1996). What is noise for the motion system? *Vision Research*, 16, 2579–2586.

Schaeffel, F. (1993). Visually guided control of refractive state: Results from animal models. In K. Simons (Ed.), *Early visual development: normal and abnormal*, 14–29 New York: Oxford University Press.

Schiller. P. H. (1985). A model for the generation of visually guided saccadic eye movements. In D. Rose and V. G. Dobson (Eds), *Models of the visual cortex*. Chichester: John Wiley and Sons.

Schneider, G. E. (1969). Two visual systems: brain mechanisms for localization and discrimination are dissociated by tectal and cortical lesions. *Science*, 163, 895–902.

de Schonen, S. and Mathivet, E. (1989). First come first served: a scenario about the development of hemispheric specialization in early infancy. *Cahiers de Psychologie Cognitive*, 9, 3–44.

Schwartz, T. L., Dobson, V., Sandstrom, D. J., and Van Hof-van Duin, J., (1987).

Kinetic perimetry assessment of binocular field size and shape in young infants. *Vision Research*, 27, 2163–2175.

Servos, P., Goodale, M. A. and Jakobson, L. S. (1992). The role of binocular vision in prehension: a kinematic analysis. *Vision Research*, 32, 1513–1521.

Shallice, T. and Burgess, P. (1996). The domain of supervisory processes and temporal organization of behaviour. *Philosophical Transactions of the Royal Society of London, Series B*, 351, 1405–1411.

Shapley, R. (1994). Linearity and non-linearity in cortical receptive fields. In G. R. Bock and J. A. Goode (Eds). *Higher order processing in the visual system: CIBA Foundation Symposium*, 184: pp. 71–87. London: CIBA Foundation.

Shapley, R. and Gordon, J. (1985). Nonlinearity in the perception of form. *Perception and Psychophysics*, 37, 84–88.

Sheliga, B. M., Riggio, L., and Rizzolatti, G. (1995). Spatial attention and eye movements. *Experimental Brain Research,* 105, 261–275.

Sheliga, B. M., Craighero, L., Riggio, L., and Rizzolatti, G. (1997). Effects of spatial attention on directional manual and ocular responses. *Experimental Brain Research*, 114, 339–351.

Sheridan, M. D. (1969). Visual screening procedures for very young children or handicapped children. In Gardiner P., Mackeith R., and Smith V. (Ed.s) *Aspects of Developmental and Paediatric Opthalmology*, 39–47, Heinemann Medical Books: London.

Sheridan, M. D. (1976). *Manual for the STYCAR vision tests*. Slough: NFER Publishing Co.

Shimojo, S., Birch, E. E., Gwiazda, J., and Held, R. (1984). Development of vernier acuity in infants. *Vision Research*, 24, 721–724.

Shipp, S. and Zeki, S. (1989). The organization of connections between areas V5 and V2 in macaque monkey visual cortex. *European Journal of Neuroscience*, 1, 333–354.

Shupert, C. and Fuchs, A. F. (1988). Development of conjugate human eye movements. *Vision Research*, 28, 585–596.

Siddiqui, A. (1995). Object size as a determinant of grasping in infancy. *Journal of Genetic Psychology*, 156, 345–348.

Sillito, A. M., Cudeiro, J., and Murphy, P. C. (1993). Orientation sensitive elements in the corticofugal influence on center-surround interactions in the dorsal lateral geniculate nucleus. *Experimental Brain Research*, 93, 6–16.

Sireteanu, R. and Rieth, C (1992). Texture segmentation in infants and children. *Behavioural Brain Research*, 49, 133–139.

Slater, A. M., Morison, V., and Somers, M (1988). Orientation discrimination and cortical function in the human newborn. *Perception*, 17, 597–602.

Sloper, J. J. (1993). Competition and co-operation in visual development. *Eye*, 7, 319–331.

Smith, J. (1989). The development of binocular vision in normal and strabismic infants. PhD. thesis, University of Cambridge.

Smith, J., Atkinson, J. Braddick, O. J., and Wattam-Bell, J. (1988). Development of sensitivity to binocular correlation and disparity in infancy. *Perception*, 17, 365.

Smith, J. C., Atkinson, J., Anker, S., and Moore, A. T. (1991). A prospective study of binocularity and amblyopia in strabismic infants before and after corrective surgery: implications for the human critical period. *Clinical Vision Sciences*, 6, 335–353.

Smyth, M. M. and Mason, U. C. (1997). Planning and execution of action in children with and without developmental coordination disorder. *Journal of Child Psychology and Psychiatry*, 38, 1023–1037.

Sokol, S. and Moskowitz, A. (1985). Comparison of pattern VEPS and preferential-looking behavior in 3-month-old infants. *Investigative Ophthalmology and Visual Science*, 26, 359–365.

Sokol, S., Hansen, V. C., Moskowitz, A., Greenfield, P., Towle, V. L. (1983). Evoked-potential and preferential looking estimates of visual acuity in pediatric patients. *Ophthalmology*, 90, 552–562.

Sokolov, E. N. (1963). *Perception and the conditioned reflex*. New York: Macmillan.

Sonksen, P. M. and Silver, J. (1988). The Sonksen-Silver Acuity System : test system and 15 page instruction manual. Windsor: Keeler Ltd.

Spelke, E. S., Breinlinger, K., Macomber, J., and Jacobson, K. (1992). Origins of knowledge. *Psychological Review*, 99, 605–32.

Spelke, E. S. and Van de Walle, G. A. (1993). Perceiving and reasoning about objects: insights from infants. In N. Eilan, R. McCarthy and B. Brewer (Eds), *Spatial representation*. Oxford: Blackwell.

Spelke, E. S. (1994). Initial Knowledge: six suggestions. *Cognition*, 50, 431–445.

Sprague, J. M. and Meikle, T. H. (1965). The role of the superior colliculus in visually guided behavior. *Experimental Neurology*, 11, 115–146.

Stiles J. and Nass, R. (1991). Spatial grouping activity in young children with congenital right and left hemisphere brain injury. *Brain and Cognition*, 15, 201–222

Stiles-Davis, J., Sugarman, S., and Nass, R. (1985). The development of spatial and class relations in four children with right hemisphere damage: Evidence for an early spatial-constructive deficit. *Brain and Cognition*, 4, 388–412.

Stryker, M., Sherk, H., Leventhal, A. G., and Hirsch, H. V. B. (1978). Physiological consequences for the cat's visual cortex of effectively restricting early visual experience with oriented contours. *Journal of Neurophysiology*, 41, 896–909

Teller, D. Y. (1979). The forced-choice preferential looking procedure: A psychophysical technique for use with human infants. *Infant Behavior and Development*, 2, 135–153.

Teller, D. Y. (1983). Measurement of visual acuity in human and monkey infants: The interface between laboratory and clinic. *Behavioural Brain Research*, 10, 15–23.

Teller, D. Y. (1997). First glances: The vision of infants. *Investigative Ophthalmology and Visual Science*, 38, 2183–2203.

Teller, D. Y. and Bornstein, M. (1987). Infant color vision and color perception. In P. Salapatek and L. Cohen (Eds), *Handbook of infant perception*, Vol. I: *From sensation to perception*. Orlando, FL: Academic Press.

Teller, D. Y. and Lindsey, D. T. (1993). Infant color vision: OKN techniques and null-plane analysis. In K. Simons (Ed.), *Early visual development: normal and abnormal*. New York: Oxford University Press.

Teller, D. Y. and Palmer, J. (1996). Infant color vision: Motion nulls for red/green-vs luminance-modulated stimuli in infants and adults. *Vision Research*, 36, 955–974.

Teller, D. Y., Morse, R., Borton, R., and Regal, D. (1974). Visual acuity for vertical and diagonal gratings in human infants. *Vision Research,* 14, 1433–1439.

Thelen, E., Corbetta, D., Kamm, K., Spencer, J. P., Schneider, K., and Zernicke, R. F. (1993) The transition to reaching: mapping intention and intrinsic dynamics. *Child Development*, 64, 1058–1098.

Thoresen, M., Penrice, U., Lorek, A., Cady, E. B., Wylezinska, M., Kirkbride, V., *et al.* (1995). Mild hypothermia after severe transient hypoxia-ischemia ameliorates delayed cerebral energy failure in the newborn piglet. *Pediatric Research*, 37, 667–670.

Tootell, R. B. H., Reppas, J. B., Malach, R., Born, R. T., Brady, T. J., Rosen, B. R., and Belliveau, J. W. (1995). Functional analysis of human MT and related visual cortical areas using magnetic resonance imaging. *Journal of Neuroscience*, 15, 3215–3230.

Trevarthen, C. B. (1974). The psychobiology of speech development. In E. H. Lenneberg (Ed.), *Language and brain: developmental aspects. Neurosciences Research Program Bulletin*, 12, 570–585.

Trevarthen, C. B. (1968). Two mechanisms of vision in primates. *Psychologische Forschung,* 31, 299–337.

Trieber, F. and Wilcox, S. (1980). Perception of 'subjective' contours by infants. *Child Development*, 51, 915–917.

Tronick, E. (1972) Stimulus control and the growth of the infant's effective visual field. *Perception and Psychophysics*, 11, 373–375.

Ungerleider, L. G. and Mishkin, M. (1982) Two cortical visual systems. In D. J. Ingle, M. A. Goodale, and R. J. W. Mansfield (Eds), *Analysis of visual behavior* (pp. 549–586). Cambridge, MA: MIT Press.

Valenza, E., Simion, F., and Umilta, C. (1994). Inhibition of return in newborns. *Infant Behavior and Development*, 17, 293–302.

Van Essen, D. C. and Maunsell, J. H. R. (1983). Hierarchical organization and functional streams in visual cortex. *Trends in Neuroscience*, 6, 370–375.

van Hof-van Duin, J., Evenhuis-Leunen, A., Mohn, G., Baerts, W., and Fetter, W. P. F. (1989). Effects of very low birth weight (VLBW) on visual development during the first year after term. *Early Human Development*, 20, 255–266.

Van Hof-van Duin, J. and Mohn, G. (1986). Visual field measurements, optokinetic nystagmus, and the threatening response: Normal and abnormal development. *Documenta Ophthalmologica Proceedings Series*, 45, 305–315.

Varner, D., Cook, J. E., Schneck, M. E., McDonald, M., Teller, D. Y. (1985). Tritan discriminations by 1- and 2-month-old human infants. *Vision Research*, 25, 821–831.

Vargha-Khadem, F. (1998). Compensation of function after hemispherectomy in childhood. *European Journal of Neuroscience*, 10, 12404.

Vital-Durand, F., Putkonen, P. T. S., and Jeannerod, M, (1974). Motion detection and optokinetic responses in dark reared kittens. *Vision Research*, 14, 141–142.

Volkmann, F. C. and Dobson, V. (1976). Infant responses of ocular fixation to moving visual stimuli. *Journal of Experimental Child Psychology*, 22, 86–99.

Watson, J. D. G., Myers, R., Frackowiak, R. S. J., Hajnal, J. V., Woods, R. P., Mazziotta, J.C., Shipp, S., and Zeki, S. (1993). Area V5 of the human brain: evidence from a combined study using positron emission tomography and magnetic resonance imaging. *Cerebral Cortex*, 3, 79–94.

Wattam-Bell, J. (1985). Analysis of infant visual evoked potentials (VEPs) by a phase-sensitive statistic. *Perception*, 14, A33.

Wattam-Bell, J. (1991). The development of motion-specific cortical responses in infants. *Vision Research*, 31, 287–297.

Wattam-Bell, J. (1992). The development of maximum displacement limits for discrimination of motion direction in infancy. *Vision Research*, 32, 621–630.

Wattam-Bell, J. (1994). Coherence thresholds for discrimination of motion direction in infants. *Vision Research*, 34, 877–883.

Wattam-Bell, J. (1995). Stereoscopic and motion Dmax in adults and infants. *Investigative Ophthalmology and Visual Science*, 36, S910

Wattam-Bell, J. (1996*a*). The development of visual motion processing. In F. Vital-Durand, O. Braddick, and J. Atkinson (Eds), *Infant vision*, pp. 79–84. Oxford University Press.

Wattam-Bell, J. (1996*b*). Visual motion processing in one-month-old infants: preferential looking experiments. *Vision Research*, 36, 1679–1685.

Wattam-Bell, J. (1996*c*). Visual motion processing in one-month-old infants: habituation experiments. *Vision Research*, 36, 1671–1677.

Wattam-Bell, J. (1996*d*). Infants' discrimination of absolute direction of motion. *Investigative Ophthalmology and Visual Science*, 37, S917.

Wattam-Bell, J., Braddick, O. J., Atkinson J., and Day, J. (1987). Measures of infant binocularity in a group at risk for strabismus. *Clinical Vision Sciences*, 1, 327–336.

Watts, C., Eyre, J. A., Kelly, S., and Ramesh, V. (1992). Development of the pincer grasp and its relationship to the development of adult corticospinal delays in man. *Journal of Physiology*, 452, P273.

Weiskrantz, L. (1986). *Blindsight: a case study and implications*. Oxford: Clarendon Press.

Werner, J. S. and Wooten, B. R. (1979). Human infant colour vision and colour perception. *Infant Behaviour and Development*, 2, 241–274.

Wertheimer, M. (1923). Untersuchung zur Lehre der Gestalt. *Psychologische Forschung*, 4, 301–350.

White, B. L., Castle, P., and Held, R. (1964). Observations on the development of visually directed reaching. *Child Development*, 35, 349–364.

Wiesel, T. N. and Hubel, D. H. (1963). Single-cell responses in striate cortex of kittens deprived of vision in one eye. *Journal of Neurophysiology*, 26, 1003–1017.

Wiesel, T. N. and Raviola, E. (1977). Myopia and eye enlargement after lid fusion in monkeys. *Nature*, 266, 66–68.

Wilson, H. R., Ferrera, V., and Yo, C (1992). A psychophysically motivated model for two-dimensional motion perception. *Visual Neuroscience*, 9, 79–97.

Wimmer, H. and Perner, J. (1983). Beliefs about beliefs: representation and constraining function of wrong beliefs in young children's understanding of deception. *Cognition*, **13**, 103–28.

Withers, S. (1996). A new clinical sign in Williams syndrome. *Archives of Disease in Childhood*, **75**, 89.

Witton, C., Talcott, J. B., Hansen, P. C., Richardson, A. J., Griffiths, T. D., Rees, A., *et al.* (1998). Sensitivity to dynamic auditory and visual stimuli predicts nonword reading ability in both dyslexic and normal readers. *Current Biology*, **8**, 791–797.

Wynn, K. (1992). Addition and subtraction by human infants. *Nature*, **358**, 749–750.

Yakovlev, P. I. and Lecours, A. (1967). The myelogenetic cycles of regional maturation of the brain. In A. Minkowski (Ed.), *Regional development of the brain in early life*. Davis: Philadelphia.

Yonas, A., Arterberry, M. E., and Granrud, C. E. (1987). Four-month olds' sensitivity to binocular and kinetic information for there-dimensional object shape. *Child Development*, **58**, 910–917.

Youdelis, C. and Hendrickson, A. (1986). A qualitative and quantitative analysis of the human fovea during development. *Vision Research*, **26**, 847–855.

Zeki, S. M. (1974). Functional organization of a visual area in the posterior bank of the superior temporal sulcus of the rhesus monkey. *Journal of Physiology*, **236**, 549–573.

Zeki, S. (1978). Functional specialization in the visual cortex of the rhesus monkey. *Nature*, **274**, 423–428.

Zeki, S. (1983*a*). The distribution of wavelength and orientation selective cells in different areas of monkey visual cortex. *Proceedings of the Royal Society of London B*, **217**, 449–470.

Zeki, S. (1983*b*). Color coding in the cerebral cortex—the reaction of cells in monkey visual cortex to wavelengths and colors. *Neuroscience*, **9**, 741–765.

Zeki, S. (1993). *A vision of the brain*. Oxford: Blackwell Scientific.

Zihl, J., von Cramon, D., and Mai, N. (1983). Selective disturbance of motion vision after bilateral brain damage. *Brain*, **106**, 313–340.

INDEX

Page number in *italics* refer to figures